The Golfer's Stroke-Saver Workout

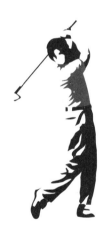

The Golfer's Stroke-Saver Workout

Thirty Minutes a Day to Longer Drives,
Lower Scores, and Better Health

ALTON SKINNER

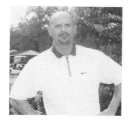
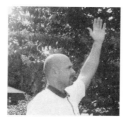
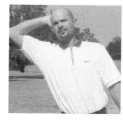
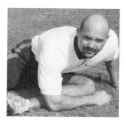
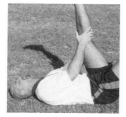
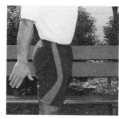
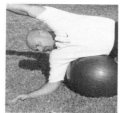
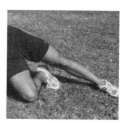

CITADEL PRESS
Kensington Publishing Corp.
www.kensingtonbooks.com

CITADEL PRESS BOOKS are published by

Kensington Publishing Corp.
850 Third Avenue
New York, NY 10022

All Kensington titles, imprints, and distributed lines are available at special quantity discounts for bulk purchases for sales promotions, premiums, fund-raising, educational, or institutional use. Special book excerpts or customized printings can also be created to fit specific needs. For details, write or phone the office of the Kensington special sales manager: Kensington Publishing Corp., 850 Third Avenue, New York, NY 10022, attn: Special Sales Department; phone 1-800-221-2647.

CITADEL PRESS and the Citadel logo are Reg. U.S. Pat. & TM Off.

First printing: April 2004

10   9   8   7   6   5   4   3   2   1

Printed in the United States of America

Library of Congress Control Number: 2003114725

ISBN 0-8065-2533-9

To all my friends, family, and coaches
who inspired me to write this book.

Acknowledgments

First and foremost, I'd like to thank everyone at Kensington Publishing, from the publisher, Laurie Parkin, and the managing director of Citadel Press, Bruce Bender, to the sales force, who have shaped this project, nurtured it, and brought it into the world. In particular, I'd like to thank my amazing editor Bob Shuman, production editor Jenna Bagnini, and copy editor Tricia Levi, who transformed this book from manuscript to a finished product. It was a pleasure working with them.

Second, I'd like to thank my agent Michael Snell. Without his help and guidance this book would not exist. From query letter to finished book. Michael was an invaluable resource. As a first time author, it was a blessing having an agent like Michael Snell to guide me through the world of publishing. I look forward to many more projects with him.

Next I owe a huge debt of gratitude to Jack Nicklaus and Gary Player. Their greatest on the golf course is only exceeded by their graciousness and generosity off the golf course.

I would like to thank all of the teachers and players who shared their valuable time and insight to improve this project. In particular I'd like to thank teachers Jim Mclean, David Pelz, Pia Nilsson, Lynn Marriot, Robert Baker, Mardell Wilkins, Annette Thompson, David Lee, Bill Maddonna, Rebecca Dengler, and Tom Patri.

Finally, I would like to thank my friends and family without their support, patience and love I do not think I would have ever started this project or finished this book.

Contents

Foreword

Tournament golf might not be considered on the same athletic plane as football, basketball, or tennis, but at the highest levels, it can be extremely demanding—physically, mentally, and emotionally—because of the amount of intense focus and concentration required. The better the player and the more often they are in contention, the greater the mental and physical exhaustion can be. Thus, the more fit a player is, the better he or she will be able to fight fatigue or exhaustion. In turn, this will keep a player sharper and more focused the deeper he or she gets into a tournament.

I have always been athletic, and grew up enjoying and competing in many different sports. But I also admit that during my twenties or my first eight years on tour, I was heavier than I should have been. I always enjoyed eating and during that time there was a greater medical acceptance of being overweight.

I knew after my first Ryder Cup in 1969, it was time to make a change. I remember being very tired after playing 36 holes on the final day, and on the flight home, I talked to my wife Barbara about the need to lose weight. I lost 20 pounds in a few weeks, and seven inches from around my hips. I remember when I returned to practicing golf. I would jog, rather than walk, between shots. I could play 18 holes in about an hour. The best part was the result. When I returned to competitive play, the new me won back-to-back tournaments.

Although it appeared as though I underwent a physical metamorphosis just prior to turning 50, I think I was just keeping up with the times and what lots of men were doing at that time. I have continued to watch my weight, dieting on and off since then.

Other than a recurring hip problem, which eventually led to a total left hip replacement surgery earlier this year, I battled occasional back problems at times during my career. Around Thanksgiving of 1988, I began a program prescribed by exercise therapist Pete Egoacue. The program and exercise were designed to keep my body functional and they probably were a major reason why I was able to avoid surgery for such a long time. I performed the exercise daily and never miss a day; I feel that if you allow yourself to miss one day, one day can easily turn to two, and so on.

I've continued to follow a daily regimen throughout my fifties certainly altering the program from time to time. Although the program allowed me to stave off hip surgery for perhaps five to six years, I made a quality-of-life decision early in 1999 and had the left hip replaced. Although my exercise regimen made the rehabilitation and recovery that much easier following the surgery, I realized once I returned to competitive play that I lacked stamina and strength. So I am currently on a program that incorporates strength training, cardiovascular work, and flexibility. Again I try to adhere to this program on a daily basis.

Without getting too detailed, I am trying to increase my aerobic capacity and increase my overall strength, particularly in my lower body, while maintaining flexibility, good posture, and balance. Five times a week I spend about 20 to 30 minutes on cardiovascular work. Three times a week I focus on strength and conditioning for about 35 minutes. We work on balance three or four times a week. And I stretch every day.

What I want to tell the golfer that currently does not exercise is the following: just look at the Senior Tour and how many players now work out on a regular basis. The most successful players on tour are the ones that work the hardest—

both on their levels of fitness and on the golf course. But isn't that true of anything in life?

If you're going to start an exercise program, make sure you have the guidance of a doctor or trained professional. And don't do too much too soon, because you not only risk injury but any setbacks can dampen your enthusiasm and motivation.

—Jack Nicklaus

Foreword

My philosophy on physical fitness is that it helps every aspect of one's life. Being physically fit gives you a strong body, a sharp mind, and good nerves, which are all vital to being a good player.

During my early twenties, I became aware of the importance of physical fitness through my association with Frank Stranahan. I started weight training during this period and while I did not worry much about my diet, I always ate a great deal of fruit, especially bananas. Since then I have become increasingly aware of the importance of diet as well as exercise. During my thirties and forties I jogged regularly and did more specific weight training, sit ups, and stretching exercises. Many of these exercises specifically were for my back and "golf muscles"— forearms, abdomen, thighs, and back. As you know, many golfers have back problems. I realize the critical importance of what we eat. I try to eat small quantities of protein, mostly fish, and concentrate on eating a lot of salads, vegetables, fruits, nuts, whole grains, and so on. Currently, I mix up my exercise program four to five times a week, which consists of sit-ups, stretching, swinging a heavy club, weight training, swimming, and power walking. Throughout my golf career, I have been helped by following the above habits, plus of course hitting thousands, if not millions of practice balls. Remember, "the harder you practice, the luckier you get!"

I feel that your physical fitness, mental state, diet, and practice are all vital to your golf game, and so is a good attitude. Our lives are filled with difficulties; it is not the problems that count but how we handle them. Count your blessings and always see the sunny side of life. A positive "can do" approach to life will greatly increase your longevity.

It is vitally important to watch your weight carefully and start exercising slowly with a program of abdominal work, stretching, and light weights. Get expert advice, like that offered in this book, on the correct methods of strengthening yourself for golf because golfers' requirements are different from other sports. This is not just for golf but if you wish to enjoy a healthy, active life with your friends and family. It's a way of life! Embrace this lifestyle.

—Gary Player

Introduction

Playing golf doesn't get you in great shape, but you need to be in great shape to play your best golf. This unique program provides a step-by-step approach to get you in the best condition to play your best golf as quickly as possible.

This program is new in that it uses simple drills to determine the exact number and type of exercise unique to your game and your body type.

The goal of this program is to prescribe the fewest possible exercises so you can devote the majority of your time playing and practicing golf and not spending all day in the gym.

I realize that you want to be a golfer who happens to work out, rather than a workout fanatic who happens to play golf.

To be in your best shape for playing golf, you don't need hours of time and tons of weight. Having consulted with top instructors like Jim McLean and Dave Pelz, and legendary players Jack Nicklaus and Gary Player, and provided fitness equipment used by Tiger Woods, I have seen what it takes for the top players to perform their best.

I want you to have access to this information. By following the Golfer's Stroke-Saver Workout, you will finally be able to train like the pros. Golf is unique among sports in that you can play the exact courses, use the exact clubs, play the exact balls, and wear the same apparel as your golfing heroes. Now you can use the same training principles your favorite tour player uses.

In chapters one and two you will test for flexibility, power, strength, and endurance. This information will reveal the precise parts of your game that you need to improve—not my game, not Tiger's game, and certainly not your regular playing partner's game—your game. One size does not fit all. Chapter three will reveal, for the first time, a quick, simple, and affordable way to find and cure your swing flaws; for example, most golfers realize the importance of stretching and flexibility, but for instance, did you know that you do not need to stretch all your muscles. A generic stretching program can actually impair your performance.

Your program may have five stretches or twenty-five stretches, but you will not have to perform one more stretch than is needed to immediately boost your performance. You will train smarter, not harder.

In chapter four you will take the strength-testing information and create a precise and detailed program of four to twelve drills that will, as Ben Hogan said, "create a powerful repeating golf swing." You will add distance to your drives, add one club length to all your irons, and become a better, more stable putter. This is the first book to provide a program to improve putting. Most other books concentrate on distance.

Remember, you drive for show and putt for dough. I had the chance to work with short-game guru Stan Utley during his days on the Buy.com tour. Utley holds the record for the fewest putts for nine holes on the PGA Tour. The record is six putts for nine holes. Stan works with a number of tour players. At the time of this writing his student Peter Jacobson had just won the Greater Hartford Open—his first tour win since 1995. Utley also has shared his training information with Jay Haas, who in 2003 is one of the hottest players on the tour at the age of 49. Putting and fitness go hand in hand if you know how to integrate them. After chapter three you will know how to do this.

In chapter five you will learn how to improve your stamina and energy on the golf course whether you ride or walk. You will learn a super short, super effective way to train your body's energy system to produce the type and kind of stamina needed for your golf game. Most cardio programs are the opposite of what is required for the sport of golf. Follow the program described here and you will avoid making the mistake common to most players, even uninformed Tour players.

Since this program is about maximizing your golf game, with the fewest exercises in the shortest time possible, chapter four will teach you how to set up a home gym. You will learn how to pick the best equipment to improve your golf game without busting your budget. What good is it to have a great golf game if you don't have money leftover to cover your greens fee?

How would you like to minimize your score and maximize your energy and power without spending one minute in the gym? Follow the eating plan outlined—the first of its kind to prescribe what to eat before, after, and during your next round of golf. For the first time you will have access to the nutritional program that results in a score three strokes lower than usual as soon as you start eating this way. Chapter seven is called "Eating for Eagles" for a reason.

Chapter eight will help you put all your new information together. Using this proven building-block approach, I promise that in 30 minutes or less per day you will play better than you ever thought you could, whether you're trying to break 80 or have won 20 majors. Just follow the Golfer's Stroke-Saver Workout and watch your scores decrease.

I want you take full advantage of this program. It will change your game, and it will change your life. But you must take action; you must follow through with this program each and every day. The workouts are brief and to the point. By taking a series of small consistent actions, you will be rewarded with powerful new habits, vibrant health, and a much improved golf game. Let's get started!

The Golfer's Stroke-Saver Workout

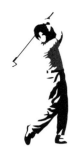

CHAPTER ONE

Your Golf Body:
Physical Demands of Golf

Tiger Woods and Justin Leonard are top-ranked golfers and have won many titles. However, Tiger is six foot two and Justin is five foot nine. This is one of the great advantages golf has over other sports. Players of different heights and body types can be successful. Tiger uses his incredible distance and looks for an opportunity to use his great power, and Justin plays small ball, using his incredible chipping and putting ability to score. What do they have in common? Their excellent training habits and physical fitness levels. In this book we will look at what it takes, besides swing technique, to become a good golfer. Players now look for any advantage and having a well-designed program is critical in reaching the top. This book will cover all aspects of complete conditioning for golf.

Fitness Demands of a Round of Golf

Researchers characterize golf as a sport in which, over the course of three to four hours, players perform brief, explosive movements with periods of long slow work in between, while maintaining a high level of mental focus. All of these characteristics, combined with maintaining proper balance and technique throughout a round, are critical for optimal performance on the links. Therefore, players must address flexibility, strength, endurance, power, body composition, and aerobic and anaerobic fitness to improve their games. What follows is a brief overview of the components of fitness for golfers. Each component will be explained more fully in later chapters.

Flexibility

Golf requires you to place your body parts in extreme ranges of motion to make a good, powerful full swing. Throughout a round you are called on to generate great force by creating a large backswing with a full turn and high arm. Strength throughout a flexible, unrestricted range of motion will prevent injury and enhance performance.

Strength and Endurance

Have your muscles ever been sore the day after you played a round of golf? If so, it's because golf requires you to have not only a good swing but also excellent strength and muscular endurance. Throughout a round, or during practice, you may hit hundreds of balls. Good muscular endurance, which means being able to apply force and sustain it over time, can help you hit the ball just as well at the end of a round or tournament as at the beginning. Also, it can prevent injuries.

Power

Golf requires explosive movements. Greater power allows you to produce a forceful swing with less effort. Players with a more powerful downswing hit the ball farther.

Optimum Body Composition

The amount of bone and water your body consists of remains constant, so you should pay attention to muscle and fat when attempting to alter body composition. You can increase the amount of muscle in the body through proper strength training and nutrition. However, it is not enough to increase muscle mass; you must also maintain an appropriate level of body fat. The two ways to affect body fat are fat-loss dieting and aerobic exercise. Fat-loss dieting, which is the correct term for a weight-loss diet because you are attempting to decrease body fat in particular, is a method of decreasing fat intake while maintaining an adequate caloric intake. Along with using fat as an energy source, aerobic exercise will improve your endurance in longer rounds and tournaments. Body fat percentages to shoot for are 8 to 18 percent for men and 15 to 25 percent for women. By following a balanced diet and including aerobic exercise in your training program, these percentages will be reached.

Anaerobic and Aerobic Fitness

What's the best way to train for golf? To answer that question, let's look at the energy demands of the sport. The energy used in a long-distance race comes from the aerobic (with oxygen) system and the energy used in short bursts of activity, such as a 20-yard dash, comes from the anaerobic (without oxygen) system. Although it is difficult to quantify the energy demand of golf, we know that it is a sport that relies on both strong aerobic and anaerobic energy systems.

The golf swing on average is less than two seconds in length. A player may expend hundreds of short bursts of energy over the course of a tournament or practice. Each swing is an anaerobic activity, so anaerobic training is important.

Does that mean you can ignore aerobic training? No! A round of golf takes three to four hours to play over miles of uneven terrain. If your aerobic fitness is low, it is difficult to recover between shots and you are likely to get tired by the end of a match. When you are tired you make mental and physical errors that result in a higher score.

Another advantage of a strong aerobic system is that it provides you with the endurance to have quality workouts.

All of these components of physical fitness are important in developing your game. To help you create an appropriate program that enhances your performance, reduces your injury risk, and increases your lifetime enjoyment in the game, start by designing a proper periodization training program.

Planning Your Conditioning Program

To reach your optimal fitness level, start by learning the demands of a round of golf and practice. Then, by designing a periodization (long-term) training program, set realistic performance goals. Tailor your training program to your individual needs, and modify them as fitness level, tournament schedule, or goals change. Each concept and activity we cover in the following chapters should fit into your periodization program. Decide which tournaments for the upcoming year are most important to you and then determine your base fitness level. Once you have identified the areas you need to focus on, use the exercises, workouts, and sample training schedules in chapters three through seven to design a customized training program for yourself. The information in chapter eight will help you prevent training injuries.

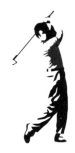

CHAPTER TWO

Your Personal Par:
Testing Golf Fitness

What makes Donna Andrews and Nancy Lopez such great golfers? Their skill level is obviously outstanding. They hit great drives and irons, and have a wonderful putting stoke. However, they not only hit the ball well, but also work hard on their physical fitness. No matter what your ability, you can't play your best golf if you are not physically fit. Being physically fit means that your heart, blood vessels, lungs, and muscles function at maximum efficiency. When you are fit, your body adjusts more easily to increased physical demands.

Fitness testing helps you monitor the effectiveness of your training program and tells you which aspects of your conditioning you need to improve. Golf fitness consists of flexibility, strength and endurance, power, agility, speed, body composition, and aerobic capacity.

Keeping track of your fitness-testing results can help you pinpoint strengths and weaknesses, design or refine a training program, and monitor your progress. From your test results, you and your coach, if you have one, can determine which fitness areas you need to improve. You can then design a specific training program based on the results. You should test at the beginning of the year and at the end of each complete program (once every three months).

You can create your profile detailing your score relative to other players of the same age and gender. Fitness testing every few months should indicate your improvement in the different categories. It will also show you where you need to modify your training program. Now let's look at each fitness component.

Flexibility Tests

Flexibility is the motion available at a joint. If a muscle cannot stretch, allowing the joint to move through a full range of motion, both injury risk and performance may be affected. Shoulder and lower back injuries are the most frequent among elite golfers. Many players have found that regular stretching can lengthen a career significantly.

Performance on the links depends mostly on your golf skill. However, having restricted flexibility may prevent you from moving efficiently, affecting the proper execution of your swing. Are you able to touch your toes without bending your knees? If not, you are like many players who have poor lower back or hamstring flexibility. Good flexibility in the hamstrings will improve torso flexibility and should decrease occurences of lower back injuries. The torso turn and hamstring stretch will indicate how much work you need in this area.

Several research studies have indicated a relationship between the loss of shoulder internal rotation and the number of years a player has competed. This loss of shoulder flexibility appears to get worse with longer periods of play. Early detection by testing your shoulder flexibility can help improve performance and reduce risk of injury.

Torso Turns

Hitting a golf ball requires a lot of turning and twisting. The key to having good flexibility is to stretch your muscles. How do you know if you are flexible enough? Take a torso turn test and see if you can get your shoulder to the center of your body. This test checks your rotator flexibility.

Procedure:

1. Sit upright in a chair with your back leaning against the backrest.

2. Place a golf club across both shoulders and wrap your arms around the club from the back so that the elbow joints and the shoulder are aligned to hold the club in place. Let your hands dangle down in front.

3. Twist your torso first to one side as far as you can while keeping your back straight. Determine the angle between your maximum reach and your original position; give yourself points accordingly.

4. Perform this test on both the right and left sides and record your turn in degrees relative to your original position.

5. Compare your scores with those in the table below.

Scoring: Torso Turns (degrees)

	Excellent	Good	Average	Needs Improvement
Right side	>90	60–90	45–60	<45
Left side	>90	60–90	45–60	<45

My score: _____

Hamstring Flexibility

Hamstring flexibility measures the amount of stretch in the muscles at the back of the thigh. This muscle is involved in maintaining a proper stance. If not properly stretched, this muscle can easily be strained or injured by the fast movements of golf.

Procedure:

1. Lie on a table with a partner stabilizing your pelvis (holding down your hip bone).

2. Raise one leg until you feel tightness in the back of the leg.

3. Have your partner measure the angle at the hip with a goniometer. A goniometer is a simple device to meas-

ure joint angles. They are available at Fitnesswhole sale.com or you also can estimate with a regular protractor. They are available for about two dollars at any office supply store.

4. Repeat on the other side.

5. Compare your scores with those in the table below.

Scoring: Hamstring Flexibility (degrees)

	Excellent	Good	Needs Improvement
Female	>85	85–75	<75
Male	>80	80–70	<70

My score: _____

Shoulder Flexibility

Shoulder flexibility describes how far you can move your arm around your shoulder joint. Adequate range of motion, both internally and externally, is essential for injury prevention and good technique during the swing. With your upper arm at a 90-degree angle to your upper body (abduction), internal rotation is when your fingers point toward your toes. External rotation is when your fingers point to your head. If the internal or external rotator muscles are tighter than they should be, imbalances and shoulder injuries are likely to occur. Many golfers have poor internal rotation.

Procedure:

1. Lie on a table with a partner stabilizing your scapula (by holding down your shoulder blade).

2. Place your upper arm at a 90-degree angle to your upper body (abduction). Bend your elbow at a 90-degree angle (pointing to the ceiling). This is considered neutral position.

3. Rotate your arm internally (fingers pointing toward toes) and externally (fingers pointing toward head), and have your partner measure both angles with a goniometer. It sounds complicated, but you simply pivot at your shoulder. Please maintain the 90° angle. This is key for a correct measurement.

4. Repeat on the other side.

5. Compare your scores with the chart below.

Scoring: Shoulder Flexibility (degrees)

	Dominant	Nondominant
Female		
External	95–105	95–105
Internal	45–55	55–65
Male		
External	90–100	90–100
Internal	40–50	50–60

My score: _____

(Same information applies for Juniors.)

Strength and Endurance Tests

Strength is the amount of weight you can lift or handle at any time. Muscular endurance is the number of times your muscles can lift a weight or how long your muscles can hold a weight.

Players are realizing that improving strength and endurance can add years to their careers and help them hit the ball farther as well.

The abdominal muscles contract every time you hit the golf ball. Sit-ups develop those muscles that are responsible for flexing or bending the trunk forward and protecting them from injury while hitting the ball.

Strength in the upper body is imperative not only to be a solid ball striker but also to prevent injuries to the shoulder, elbow, and wrist. Push-ups will indicate overall shoulder, chest, and tricep strength, and the grip-strength measurement can show not only forearm strength but also differences between the dominant and nondominant sides.

Sit-ups

We all know that it is important to have strong legs to carry you over the course and maintain proper position in the swing, and that you need strong arms to provide a forceful swing. Equally, if not more important, are your abdominal and lower back muscles. These muscles serve as a link between the upper and lower body as you transfer force from the ground all the way up to the club. For training purposes, you may wish to perform crunches to reduce strain on your hip flexors and lower back. However, for testing purposes, I always recommend that someone hold your feet while you perform a complete sit-up. Sit-ups test your abdominal strength and endurance.

Procedure:

1. Lie on your back with your knees flexed at 90 degrees.
2. Have a partner hold your feet so they do not move while you perform the sit-ups.
3. Cross your arms over your chest and place your hands on opposite shoulders.
4. Perform as many sit-ups as possible in a 60-second period (have your partner count and keep an eye on the clock).
5. To count as a complete sit-up, the elbows must touch the knees in the up position, while keeping the arms against the body, and the shoulder blades must touch the mat in the down position, with the hips touching the mat.
6. Compare your score to those in the following table.

Scoring: Sit-ups (number completed in one minute)

	Excellent	Good	Average	Needs Improvement
Female				
Adult	>53	46–53	42–45	<42
Male				
Adult	>58	51–58	47–50	<47
Juniors	>63	56–63	50–55	<50

My score: _____

Push-ups

Push-ups measure your upper body strength and endurance.

Procedure:

1. Get in a prone position with hands shoulder-width apart and the weight of your lower body on your toes.

2. Extend your arms but keep your head, shoulders, back, hips, knees, and feet in a straight line.

3. Have a partner record the number of push-ups you complete in a 60-second period; if you stop before sixty seconds, count the number up to the time you stop.

4. To count as a complete push-up, the upper arm must reach parallel to the floor or below in the down position, the arms must be completely extended in the up position, and you must maintain straight body alignment.

5. Compare your score with those in the following table.

Scoring: Push-ups (number completed in one minute)

	Excellent	Good	Average	Needs Improvement
Female				
Adult	>44	34–44	27–33	<27
Junior	>42	34–42	20–33	<20
Male				
Adult	>52	49–52	35–48	<35
Junior	>49	40–49	30–39	<30

My score: _____

Power Test

Power is the amount of work you can perform in a given period. Power is needed during activities using both strength and speed. Improving either or both of these fitness components can help your athleticism tremendously. Lower body power helps you transfer energy quickly; upper body power helps you hit the ball throughout the round.

Medicine Ball Toss

Training with a medicine ball can be practical because you can mimic the golf swing. Tossing the medicine ball involves the whole body. There is a strong relationship between performing well in these tests and overall fitness in golfers. Pay particular attention to the technique of the tosses. Proper technique will involve knee flexion and extension and a significant amount of trunk rotation, not a toss with the arms only. The medicine ball toss is a measure of power.

Procedure:

1. Stand at a designated spot facing forward and hold a six-pound medicine ball in your right hand.

2. Take one step and toss the ball, simulating the down-swing. Stay behind the line.

3. Measure the distance from the line to the place where the ball landed.

4. Repeat for the left side.

5. Compare your scores with those in the tables below.

6. Repeat above steps for the Backswing toss.

Scoring: Downswing Medicine Ball Toss (feet)

	Excellent	Good	Average	Needs Improvement
Female				
Adult	>30.5	25–30.5	19.5–24	<19.5
Junior	>32	26–32	20–25	<20
Male				
Adult	>39	32–39	25–31	<25
Junior	>42	35–42	28–34	<28

My score: _____

Scoring: Backswing Medicine Ball Toss (feet)

	Excellent	Good	Average	Needs Improvement
Female				
Adult	>30	24–30	17.5–23.5	<17.5
Junior	>31	25–31	18–24	<18
Male				
Adult	>37.5	30.5–37.5	23.5–30	<23.5
Junior	>42	34–42	26–33	<26

My score: _____

The overhead and reverse overhead tosses use the same muscles as the swing. You will be most successful if you use ground reaction force properly. From physics we know that for every reaction there is an equal and opposite force. Releasing the medicine ball at a 45-degree angle will give you the best results. Both overhead and reverse tosses are measures of power.

Procedure (Overhead):

1. Stand at a designated spot facing forward and hold a six-pound medicine ball.

2. Take one step and toss the ball from an overhead position while staying behind the line.

3. Measure the distance from the line to the place where the ball landed.

4. Compare your scores with those in the table below.

Scoring: Overhead Medicine Ball Toss (feet)

	Excellent	Good	Average	Needs Improvement
Female				
Adult	>22.5	18.5–22.5	14.5–18	<14.5
Junior	>23	19–23	15–18	<15
Male				
Adult	>30.5	25.5–30.5	20–25	<20
Junior	>34	29–34	23–28	<23

My score: _____

Procedure (Reverse Overhead):

1. Stand at a designated spot and hold a six-pound medicine ball with both hands.

2. Using an underhand position, toss the ball behind you as far as possible.

3. Measure the distance from the line to the place where the ball landed.

4. Compare your scores with those in the table below.

Reverse Medicine Ball Toss (feet)

	Excellent	Good	Average	Needs Improvement
Female				
Adult	>32.5	26.5–32.5	20.5–26	<20.5
Junior	>34	27–34	20–26	<20
Male				
Adult	>43.5	35–43.5	27–34.5	<27
Junior	>46	38–46	31–37	<31

My score: _____

Body Composition Test

Knowing your body composition is the result of measuring, through various methods, the percentages of fat, muscle, bone and water that your body is made of. The percentage of body fat gives a good indication of your physical condition. Percentages to shoot for are listed in the table on page 18.

Body fat can be measured in a variety of ways. The quick method is more accurate and cost-effective than other methods. It provides a simple non-invasive method of estimating body fat.

Procedure (for men; women require a different formula):

1. Determine your total body weight and multiply it by 1.082 (men's weight constant and add 94.420 to the product).

    a. My weight _____ × 1.082 = _____ + 94.420 = _____

2. Take your waist measurement at the belly button and multiply by 4.150 (the men's waist constant).

    b. My waist _____ × 4.150 = _____

3. Subtract waist factor (b) from weight factor (a) to determine Lean Body Mass (LBM).

    (b) _____ minus (a) _____ = _____ (LBM)

4. Take your total body weight and subtract your lean body mass (LBM) to determine your body fat.

    My weight _____ minus LBM _____ = _____ body fat

5. Take your body fat and multiply it by 100, then divide the product by your body weight. The result is your body fat percentage.

    My body weight × 100 = _____ divided by body fat =

    _____

    My percentage of body fat is _____

6. Take body fat percentage and subtract it from 100 percent. The difference is your lean body percentage.

    (100) minus your body fat _____ = _____ (lean body mass percentage)

Women's Body Composition Test

1. Determine your total body weight and multiply it by 0.732 (women's weight constant one) and add 8.987 (women's weight constant two). This is your weight factor.

    a. My weight _____ × 0.732 = _____ + 8.987 = _____

2. Take your wrist measurement and divide it by 3.140 (the women's wrist constant). The result is your wrist factor.

   b. My wrist measurement _____ divided by 3.140 = _____

3. Take your abdominal measurement (at the belly button) and multiply it by 0.157 (the women's abdominal constant). The result is your abdominal factor.

   c. My abdominal measurement _____ × 0.157 = _____

4. Take your hip measurement and multiply it by 0.249 (the women's hip constant). The result is your hip factor.

   d. My hip measurement _____ × 0.249 = _____

5. Take your forearm measurement and multiply it by 0.434 (the women's forearm constant). The result is your forearm factor.

   e. My forearm measurement _____ × 0.434 = _____

6. Take your weight factor (a) and add your wrist factor (b), subtract your abdominal factor (c), subtract your hip factor (d), and add your forearm factor (e). The result is your lean mass.

   f. My weight factor _____ + my wrist factor _____

      − my abdominal factor _____ − my hip factor _____

      + my forearm factor _____ = my Lean Body Mass

7. Take your total body weight and subtract your lean body mass. The result is your body fat.

   g. My body weight _____ − my lean body mass _____

      = _____

8. Take your body fat and multiply it by 100 and divide the product by your total body weight.

    h. My body fat _____ × 100 + _____ divided by my

        total body weight _____ = _____

9. Take your body fat percentage and subtract it from 100 percent. The result is your lean body mass percentage.

    i. 100 percent – my body fat percentage _____ = _____

Body Composition (suggested ranges for golfers)

	Female	Male
Adult	15–25%	8–20%
Junior	12–22%	5–15%

My Score: _____

Aerobic Endurance Test

Aerobic endurance is the ability to take in, transport, and use oxygen. Aerobic energy is used during prolonged, steady, paced activities, mainly using the large muscle groups. Examples of activities include jogging, cycling, and swimming.

Aerobic endurance is important in golf. When you become aerobically fit you can remain focused longer and more easily and perform longer without becoming tired. As your endurance improves, your ligaments and tendons will become tougher, reducing the threat of injury and laying the foundation for more intense training.

One accurate and simple test to measure your aerobic fitness is the one-and-a-half-mile run. Although golf is performed at a slow speed, a round lasts four to five hours and covers a distance of four to five miles on average. This time and distance are taxing on your aerobic system. When completing the one-and-a-half-mile distance, you should focus on running at a consistent pace through all six laps. You should train for longer distances in the off-season and preseason.

Procedure:

1. Stand at the start finish line on a level 440-yard track.
2. Have a partner give the command, "ready, go" and start the stopwatch.
3. Complete one-and-a-half miles (six laps) and record your score.
4. Compare your score with those in the table below.

1.5-Mile Run (minutes:seconds)

	Excellent	Good	Average	Needs Improvement
Female				
Adult	<11:49	11:49–13:43	13:44–15:08	>15:08
Junior	<10:30	10:30–11:00	11:01–11:30	>11:30
Male				
Adult	<8:44	8:44–10:47	10:48–12:20	>12:20
Junior	<9:45	9:45–10:15	10:16–11:00	>11:00

My score: _____

Golf Fitness Package

Many factors contribute to success in golf and because the game is based on skill, just being strong or fast does not make you a better player than someone else. However, you can always improve your physical abilities and address your weaknesses. Top players are constantly looking for an edge over their opponents. They can strike the ball well, so proper fitness training may make the difference in putting them ahead of the competition. Why wouldn't you test yourself on these fitness components like the pros do? Keeping track of fitness-testing results can help you track your performance, reduce the risk of injury, and develop a better understanding of your fitness abilities. You can then design proper training programs as outlined in *The Golfer's Stroke-Saver Workout.*

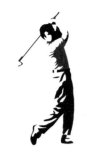

CHAPTER THREE

Stretching Your Drives:
Warm-up and Flexibility

How would you like to instantly improve your golf game? How would you like to increase your clubhead speed and reduce your score without changing your equipment or exercise program. If you are like most of my clients you answered yes. When working with the Duke University women's golf team I discovered that an intergraded warm-up program could create immediate positive changes in performance on the course. Now you can follow the same program they used during the research. Remember a quality conditioning program for golf includes strength, flexibility, and endurance training. If any component of a golfer's training program is neglected, players are unlikely to achieve their full potential and are more susceptible to injury while playing. Golf demands proper warm-up and flexibility training for all areas of the body.

The **standard warm-up** for all Golfer's Stroke-Saver Workout workouts consist of the following three parts:

1. **General warm-up:** raises your body temperature and respiration. It consists of at least five minutes of an aerobic activity like jogging or bicycling. It does not matter which aerobic activity you choose so long as you break a sweat.

2. **Specific warm-up:** prepares the muscles that receive the most stress while playing golf, especially the shoulder muscles and lower back. Because the shoulder is so complex, you must perform several exercises for it.

Heavy weights are not necessary; just be certain to get a full range of motion in each exercise.

3. **Back, shoulder, and wrist/forearm stretches:** develop and maintain flexibility in those areas. For best results, perform these stretches after you have thoroughly prepared your back and shoulders with the general and specific warm-ups.

Warm-Up Exercises

Shoulder Clocks

This exercise is an excellent way to warm up the biggest joint in the shoulder complex. The complex consists of the shoulder blade and the connection to the rib cage. This is important

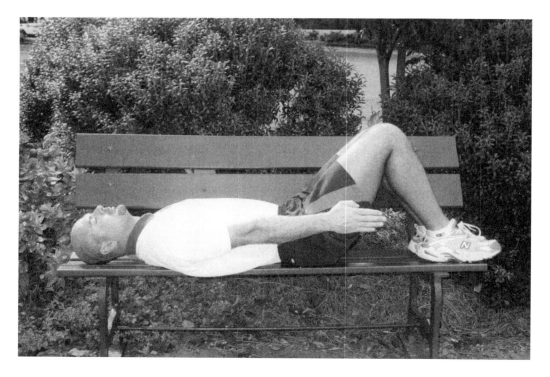

shoulder clocks start

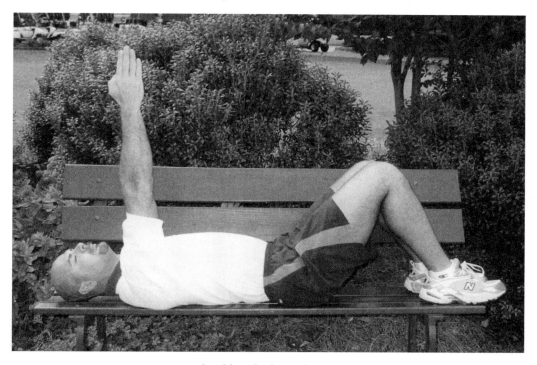

shoulder clocks mid point

to include in your warm-up so you can minimize any chance of shoulder pain caused by your golf swing.

This drill can be performed either standing or lying on your back. Once you have regained your coordination and mastered how to perform this drill, you will get good results quickly when the drill is performed standing.

- Lie on your back with your knees bent comfortably.
- Pretend that your shoulder is a hand on a clock. Toward your ear is 12 o'clock, toward your hips is 6 o'clock. Forward is 9 o'clock and in the opposite direction is 3 o'clock.
- Alternate moving your shoulder between 12 and 6 o'clock five times and then between 3 and 9 o'clock five times.
- Repeat with your other shoulder.

- After performing on each shoulder, attempt to hit each number on the clock in turn. Perform in the clockwise and counterclockwise directions five times on each of your shoulders.

Hip Rotations

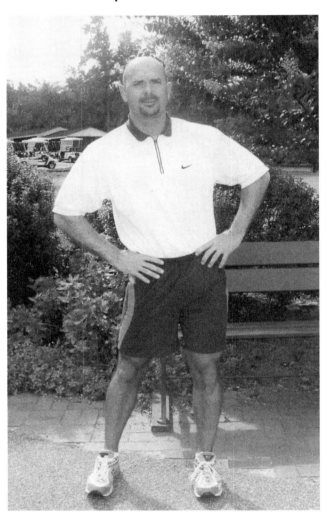

hip rotations

Your hips are composed of ball and socket joints. To warm up these joints for golf, do the following:

- Place your hands on your hips above your pockets. With your feet shoulder-width apart, begin to rotate your pelvis in circles, starting small and progressively getting larger.

- Increase the size of the circles, from small to large, as possible, over 12 to 15 repetitions.

- Reverse the direction of movement and do another 12 to 15 rotations.

Weight Shifting

Weight shifting requires you to perform a much more golf-specific movement pattern than the previous hip rotations. This drill is used to warm up the sacroiliac and pubic joints of the pelvis. They are key to a full swing. You also will warm up the muscles of your pelvis, including your hip rotators and adductors.

- Put your hands on your hips at your pockets. As you shift your weight toward one leg, allow your other knee to drop downward and inward slightly; this unlocks your sacroiliac joint on that side and frees your pelvis so it rotates more easily.

- Start with small movements and gradually increase your movements to full weight shift and pelvic rotation by the tenth repetition on each side. When you get to the last two repetitions on each side, your weight shift should be about 80 percent stance leg to 20 percent trailing leg.

Foot and Ankle Warm-up

Ankle rotations are key for preparing to drive the ball and shots from the rough.

- Place your hands on your hips and begin to shift your weight left and right. As you shift to your left, let the arch of your left foot get large and allow your foot to roll so the weight is on the outside of your left foot and the inside of your right foot.

- Alternate from side to side, letting your ankles rotate and your feet transfer the weight from the outside to the inside of your feet.

- Perform 10 times on each side.

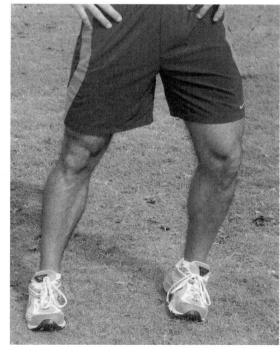

foot and ankle warm-up

Your ankle works best as a hinge joint, but your golf swing requires your ankle to actually rotate as part of a sequence of movements in related joints. Warming up your ankles is very important if you have a stiff back, hips, or shoulders, because this limitation will cause excessive movement at your ankles as a way to compensate.

Arm and Leg Flicks

The Arm Flick drill is performed by flicking your arm in a relaxed swinging motion, as though you were trying to flick something sticky off your fingers. Leg Flicks are done by standing on one leg and flicking your free leg, as though trying to flick pebbles out of your shoe. Arm and leg flicks relax the muscles crossing all the joints of your legs and arms.

- Rhythmically flick each arm and leg 20 times, progressing from mild to moderate speed. This will minimize compensation, faulty muscle recruitment patterns, and inconsistency in your swing.

Swing Progressions

Swing progressions are the final stage of your warm-up for the best golf.

- Take a seven iron and perform ten half-swings at 50-percent effort.
- After a short rest perform five full swings, increasing your effort with each swing from 50-percent speed to full speed.
- For your final exercise, swing your driver ten times, progressively increasing to full swing speed and power by your tenth swing.

You are now ready to play the best golf your body is capable of playing. A quality warm-up is a quick and powerful way to boost your on-course performance. If you follow only this

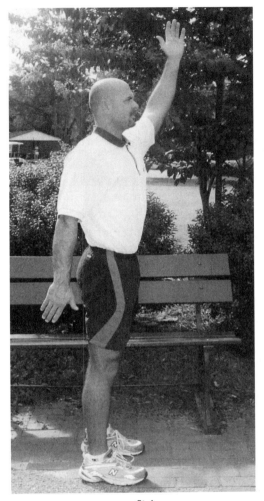

arm flick

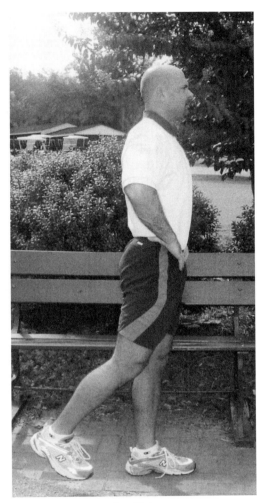

leg flick

warm-up program, I promise you will play better golf. But if you really wish to enhance your game you must follow a personalized stretching program. This program is custom and relies on a minimum of drills to improve your game. My goal is to provide the shortest training possible so that you have the maximum amount of time available for playing and golf-skill practice. Are you ready to start playing your best golf? Let's create your program.

Recognizing the critical role of flexibility in peak performance and injury prevention the Golfer's Stroke-Saver Workout has put together recommendations for a flexibility training program. Flexibility needs are specific to each individual.

You can use tests that measure flexibility to identify areas where improved flexibility is needed and to demonstrate progress in a specific flexibility program. An example of an appropriate test for flexibility is the torso turn and hamstring flexibility test.

In many instances in this chapter we include more than one flexibility exercise for each body part because some exercises are more basic than others. If one area of the body has limited range of motion, you may want more than one stretching exercise for that body segment. Once you can perform one stretch, you may want a more advanced stretch for that area. It is recommended that a player focuses on areas of the body that have the most limited flexibility. Do not just stretch the areas that are more flexible or easiest to stretch. This will take time from other areas that need special attention and may decrease joint stability or promote imbalances.

The following drills will determine precisely the muscles, unique to you, that must be stretched to restore balance to your golf swing.

Neck Bend

- Stand or sit in front of a mirror and bend your neck as if you are trying to touch your ear to your shoulder. Make sure you do not dip your shoulder downward as you bend your neck and head. Your normal range of motion should be between 24 to 40 degrees.

If you are able to bend one side much more than the other, you need only stretch the tight side. Stretch twice a day for two weeks. If you do not improve, it may be prudent to consult with a physical therapist, chiropractor, or a related medical professional.

Neck Turn

- Sit upright in a chair, keeping good upright posture with your shoulders and back against your chair. Turn your head to your right and then to the left. Determine how far you turn.

Your normal range of turn should be 70 to 90 degrees on both sides. Ideal rotation is when you can turn your head until your chin lines up directly with your shoulder. If you are over sixty years old, 70 degrees is the normal amount of turn for you.

If you can't turn your head between these ranges, use the Neck Turn Stretch prior to your round and in your developmental stretching program.

When your neck is tight, it is very likely that you will take your eyes off the ball during your backswing. This can cause you to lose your swing plane and/or have a poor clubface angle at impact.

Sweetheart

This drill determines if the muscles that lift your shoulder toward your ear will restrict your neck rotation because of being short or tight. You will need the results from the Neck Turn test to determine your range of motion.

- Place one arm around a partner, make sure you completely relax your arm and shoulder. Turn your head away from the arm on your friend's shoulder. Switch arms and do the same on the other side. You should be able to turn your neck the same range as you did during the Neck Turn drill.

If you have less movement on either side with this drill, your levator scapulae muscle needs to be lengthened.

If you are tight in this area your shoulder girdle will not be able to rotate around your spine and rib cage. This tightness will reduce your left neck rotation during the backswing, which can cause you to lose sight of the ball. If you are tight in this area you will have unwanted compression in your neck when you move your arms. This will often appear in the form of a tension headache and/or pain in your neck after play or practice. If you are tight in this area make sure to stretch it prior to play or practice.

Scratch

This drill is used to measure internal and external rotation of your shoulders.

- This is a two-stage drill: first, reach over your shoulder and try to touch the top inside corner of the opposite shoulder blade to determine your external rotation; second, reach behind your back and try to touch the lower part of your opposite shoulder blade. This will show your level of internal rotation.

The farther your fingers are from your shoulder blade, the tighter you are. To correct this tightness, you will use the Lateral Shoulder Rotator stretch if tight externally or the Medial Shoulder Rotator stretch for internal tightness.

If your right shoulder has limited external rotation, your follow-through will be restricted. If it is your left shoulder then your backswing will be restricted. If you experience tightness in your left external rotators then you are likely to lose your swing axis and also be forced to alter your swing path.

Chest

Your chest is made up of two muscles, the pectoralis major and minor.

- To measure your level of tightness, lay flat on your back on the floor with your hands behind your head. Let your arms drop to the floor.

You should be able to lay both forearms flat on the floor. If one or both of the forearms fail to reach the floor, then your chest is tight and needs to be stretched.

If you are tight in this area you will have a combination of the swing faults caused by tight neck muscles and tight shoulder muscles. Loss of swing axis, an altered swing path, and inability to keep your eye on the ball during the backswing can happen with tight pecs. You also should know that this condition may cause or increase your risk of shoulder looseness, impingement syndrome, and instability, which can cause pain during your backswing or follow-through.

Spine Turn

Lay flat on your back with you knees in the air at right angles. Slowly lower you legs to one side. You should be able to drop your legs flat on the floor without your opposite shoulder coming off the floor. The greater the distance your legs are from the floor when your opposite shoulder begins to lift, the less spinal rotation you have.

When you are limited in your spinal rotation you will tend to shift and sway with your hips during the backswing and follow-through. Often you may overuse your shoulder to compensate for the lack of a full turn. When your spine can't fully rotate, your coil, the source of power in the swing, is limited. To compensate for the lack of a coil, you may try to accelerate the club with your arms, a common cause of elbow pain. You may also have faults related to swing path, clubface angle at impact, and maintaining your swing axis. Use the Trunk Rotation to improve your spinal rotation.

Hip Flexor

Lie down on a sturdy table or firm bed. Position yourself so that both of your legs are dangling off the end of the table and not touching the floor. Put one hand under your back, directly beneath your belly button. With your other hand, bring your knee to your chest until you feel your spine start to press down on your hand. Look down to see if your opposite leg has lifted off of the table. Also, notice whether your lower leg is hanging straight down toward the floor.

If your thigh on the table stays flat and your lower leg stays at a right angle to the floor then you have optimal flexibility in this area. However, if your thigh comes off the table, you will need to use the Hip Flexors stretch. If your lower leg does not hang straight toward the floor then you will use the Swiss Ball Quadriceps Stretch (25).

If your hip flexors are short then you may be limited in your backswing because of a reduced ability to turn your trunk. This reduces distance off the tee. You may also have a limited follow-through, reducing your ability to hit the ball straight and robbing you of distance.

Short hip flexors contribute to back pain. Short hip flexors are the most common cause of muscle imbalance, sometimes causing your lower abdominals and hamstrings to lengthen and weaken as your lower back muscles become shorter and tighter with your hip flexors. This imbalance leads to many golfers suffering from low back pain.

Lower Hamstring

Lie on the floor with both of your legs extended. Place one hand under your back directly beneath your belly button. Lift one leg, slightly bent at the knee, until it is perpendicular (90 degrees) to the floor until you feel your spine start to press down on your hand. If you have normal hamstring length you should be able to straighten your leg to 170 degrees. If you can't do this then you need to improve your hamstring flexibility.

Your posture at address is frequently affected by short, tight hamstrings. As your hamstrings become short, your pelvis can not rotate forward to keep a proper working relationship with your spine. This causes excessive forward bending of your lower back and often your entire spine. When your lower back and/or mid-back are forced to bend more than normal because of short hamstrings, your turn (spine rotation) is reduced. Reduced rotation limits your ability to fully coil and you will reduce your distance off the tee. Often you may begin to swing with your arms, which will create the same swing flaws as reduced spinal rotation (see Medicine Ball Toss test, p. 25).

Upper Hamstring

This will determine the length of your upper hamstrings and the ability to allow normal motion at your hips.

Pinch a bit of skin at your lower back directly opposite your belly button. Hold your other arm at a right angle to your side. You should be able to bend forward 50 degrees while holding on to the bit of skin and keeping the normal curve in your lower back. Should you bend less than the ideal amount, use this drill as the corrective stretch Standing Hamstring Stretch (22). Tight upper hamstrings produce the same flaws as tight lower hamstrings.

Internal and External Hip Rotation

Stand against a wall with your feet hip-width apart. Slowly rotate your leg outward by pivoting on your heel. Make sure your pelvis does not move and that your leg is locked. This measures internal rotator length. To measure external rotator length, simply rotate the same leg inward in the same manner. Be sure your pelvis is square to the front and not turning outward.

Normal internal rotators will allow your foot to turn outward to at least 45 degrees; normal external rotators will allow you to turn the leg 40 degrees from the starting point.

Tight hip rotators limit your backswing and follow-through. This will cause overuse of the shoulders and back during the swing. Imbalance at the hips is a common contributor to overuse injuries to your back, shoulders, and elbows. Senior players should pay a lot of attention to this test, since tight hips lead to low back pain and a loss of power.

Tight hip rotators cause the swing faults such as loss of swing path, loss of swing arc, and overuse of your arms and wrist. To lengthen your hip rotators you will use the External and Internal Hip Rotators stretches (18, 19).

Side Bend

Stand with your feet together and your heels, back, and head pressed against a wall. Keep your head, shoulders, and back against the wall as you slide your hand down the right leg. Go as far as you can without your left heel lifting off the ground. Avoid sticking your hips out to the left or right.

You should be able to reach your knees on both sides. If you are not even on both sides use the Oblique Abdominals stretch (13) on the tight side.

It is common to find that if you are tight on this test you also were tight on the Spine Turn. You cannot do one motion without the other taking place at the same time. So, a tight side bend will also cause a limited turn, excessive sway during the take away and follow-through, loss of swing path, incorrect clubface angle at impact, loss of swing axis, and shoulder compensation with a limited body coil.

Arm Raise

Stand with your heels one foot from the wall, and your back, buttocks, and head against the wall. Have a friend place his hand between the wall and your lower back to see how much curve you have at this position. Lift your arms toward the wall, then have your friend check your lower back curve.

You should be able to lift your arms to the wall without your lower back moving away from the wall. If you can't, this reveals tight latissimus dorsi muscles. Use the Latissimus Dorsi stretch (11) to correct this shortened back muscle.

Shortened lats will change your backswing and follow-through. If your lat is short and begins to become overly stimulated it can overpower the external rotation of your shoulder. This causes you to close the clubface at impact. Whether you hook or slice depends on what changes you made to your swing path on the way down.

Torso Extension

Start with your heels one foot from the wall and your back, buttocks, and head against the wall. If your mid-back does not extend enough and you cannot place your head against the wall, you need to improve your torso extension. If you can lift your arms with your buttocks, back, and head against the wall, then you have normal torso extension. If your spine does not flatten, then you are at risk for a shoulder injury.

You need good extension to protect your shoulder joint from impingement or overloading as you bring it across your body during the backswing. With a restricted backswing you reduce your power and distance.

Your body will compensate for tightness in this area by creating excessive movements in your shoulders and extending your hips during the backswing. The excessive movement of your shoulders leads to swinging just with the arms, which leads to shoulder injuries. Players also tend to come off their swing axes when they lack torso extension, which changes both the swing path and swing arc. This results in a chopping swing with fat, thin, and inconsistent shots.

The Foam Roller and Longitudinal Mobilizations stretches (28 and 29) will help correct this area; single-arm dumbbell rows will help to improve torso extension.

Press-up

This test determines if you can bend your back properly and how well your lumbar disk is working.

Lie face down on the floor with your hands beside the top of your shoulders. Take a deep breath in and begin to press up your upper body like you are doing a push-up; keep your hips on the floor. Exhale as you lift up. Make sure you relax your buttocks and back muscles. By exhaling on the way up it makes the movement easier.

Ideally, you will be able to straighten your arms and keep your hips on the floor.

The more bend in your arms as your hips lift up, the tighter your lumbar spine. You should use the Press-up (27) in your corrective stretching program. This exercise is designed to restore normal motion in your lumbar spine, not to make the muscles stronger.

If you lack lumbar extension you won't have an optimal backswing or follow-through. You may overuse your shoulders to compensate, leading to impingement syndrome. This is when you have pain in your right shoulder at the end of the backswing and/or pain in your right shoulder during the follow-through.

Note: If you experience restrictions while doing the Press-up or Torso Turn, it is important to have a doctor check for spinal arthritis. Before trying the Press-up and Foam Roller and Longitudinal Mobilizations stretches, get it checked. If you have arthritis in your spine some of your vertebrae may be fused together. Caution: If you perform these drills as a means to reach normal range of motion with this condition, you may fracture your spine. Get medical clearance to do these drills.

The Best Stretches for Golf Flexibility and Swing Mechanics

Now that you have identified exactly which areas are hampering your swing you can develop your stretching program. Now it is time to pick the best stretches to improve your flexibility and swing mechanics. First, include the stretches listed in the chart for the areas your flexibility test revealed as being tight. Second, turn to and review the table that lists the 28 most common swing faults (see page 69), find your most common faults, and add the stretches listed to your routine. It's that easy! Now you have a program that contains no more and no less stretches than you need to develop a correct, powerful, repeating golf swing.

This systematic approach, following a fundamentally correct progression, is the quickest and most efficient way to improve your golf swing. By performing a combination of these stretches you are well on your way to correcting your body and swing faults. You will use these stretches in your developmental stretch program until your swing fault is corrected. Once corrected, you can move on to a maintenance program to keep this fault from coming back.

Developmental Stretching Program

Muscle imbalances and limited movement in your joints may be responsible for your swing flaws. It is time to start a developmental stretching program, which will lengthen your tight muscles and is essential to play injury-free golf. When you do anything that changes the length of your muscles and/or the balance between your muscles, your nervous system will compensate for these changes. Over time, this compensation will cause you to develop improper movement patterns in your swing and can lead to injury while playing or training.

Maximizing Your Stretching Program

To get the most from your program you should stretch at two key times:

1. **Before Play, Practice, and Training.** This will create improved range of motion and, therefore, improved technique. It is important to only stretch your short, tight muscles.

2. **Before Going to Sleep.** You must take the time to stretch your muscles one to two hours before going to sleep. After work, exercise, or golf your muscles will become slightly shorter and tighter as a reaction to being fatigued from your physical efforts. If you fail to lengthen your muscles before sleep your muscles will progressively shorten and tighten. This happens because your body does most of its healing and recovery while you sleep. By stretching before going to sleep you maximize your improvement by restoring your muscles to their proper length during the healing process.

Maintaining Improved Flexibility

Once you have restored balance to your body by following your stretching and strengthening exercises, you have to maintain the improvements. Your maintenance program will focus on your problem areas and the muscles you use most when you swing the golf club. Even if you feel loose, you must continue to stretch. Even if your assessment revealed you to be flexible enough for golf, over time through work, golf, exercising, and so on you will develop muscle imbalances if you are not careful. To keep this from happening, stretch regularly by following a maintenance stretching program that consists of:

Hip Flexors (15)

Lumbar Erectors (16)

90/90 Hip Stretch (17)

Rocking Groin Stretch (21)

Lying Hamstring Stretch (23)

Upper Traps (3)

Medial Shoulder Rotators and Chest (5)

Lateral Shoulder Rotators (6)

Latissimus Dorsi (11)

Trunk Rotation (14)

Pre-Round Stretching

Many players do not have enough flexibility to have a correct, powerful, repeating golf swing. Work, old injuries, and your current aches and pains may cause you to become tight even after following your developmental or maintenance program in a matter of hours. Because of this you must perform a pre-round stretching and warm-up program, which should include muscle-mobilization drills.

To maximize your success during play and practice you must stretch and warm up before you start. But you must warm up and stretch properly. If you use the wrong method of stretching on the wrong muscles, your risk of injury will increase. This is a terrible mistake most players make: for example, if you use the traditional extended stretch method (Static Stretching) to stretch your tight muscles you will cause your muscles to relax. You don't want your muscles to relax, especially those that hold your joints in place. Here's why: Scientists believe that your body stores movement patterns in your brain. You have a huge variety of movement skills and abilities stored as general-movement patterns. A general-movement pattern is a set routine of movements similar to other patterns of movement. Take chipping, driving, or pitching; each of these swings requires your brain to use the "Trunk Rotation" pattern or a movement pattern that has the same tempo as your golf swing. From this point, your brain adjusts the particular variables like speed, intensity, and timing to produce a certain swing based on the current conditions.

If you have used static stretching with extended holding of the stretch position, as most players have been taught to use as part of their warm-up, your muscles will lengthen without your brain being able to effectively gauge how much the length of your muscle has changed; for example, if you were to go out to the range and drive the ball after using static stretching, your brain would instantly notice that the input from your muscles that you use to drive the ball does not match the information stored as the "trunk rotation-golf swing-driver pattern." This causes your brain to try to alter your swing to match the pattern stored in your brain as your "ideal driver swing pattern" because of the sudden change in your body's movement ability.

Here's the problem: this process of adjustment often takes longer than the time between your backswing and follow-through. I am sure you have experienced situations in which you take your club back and on the way down to impact you sense that something was wrong in your swing, but you couldn't adjust in time. If your muscles are not properly controlled by your nervous system because of using the wrong stretching method you will reduce your swing consistency and increase your risk of injury out on the course.

The Best Way to Perform Your Pre-Round Stretches

When you stretch before play or practice do not hold your stretch position for more than one to two seconds. The best way to warm up is to use dynamic stretching. This method of stretching requires you to constantly move from one stretch position to another without stopping. You move from the stretch to relaxed muscle position repeatedly until you loosen up.

Remember never to move too quickly or to stop moving for more than one to two seconds. Since you are constantly moving your brain will constantly monitor the changing length of your muscles. This keeps your joints from becoming destabilized or reducing your coordination as compared to static stretching.

The Best Way to Perform Your Post-Round Stretches

Stretching after your round is an ideal way to limit your muscle soreness. As your muscles tire, they tighten and blood flow to them is reduced. Also, after a long round of golf or practice, your metabolism remains elevated for several hours. During this period, your muscles continue to produce acidic waste products that can irritate your nerve endings. This causes your muscles to tighten even more. Post-round stretching will prevent muscle soreness after your round of golf.

Your post-round stretching program will consist of stretches that target the muscles you use the most during your golf swing. These are:

Hip Flexors (15)

Lumbar Erectors (16)

90/90 Hip Stretch (17)

Rocking Groin Stretch (21)

Lying Hamstring Stretch (23)

Upper Traps (3)

Medial Shoulder Rotators and Chest (5)

Lateral Shoulder Rotators (6)

Latissimus dorsi (11)

Trunk Rotation (14)

Important: Post-round stretching does not replace your developmental or maintenance stretching program. Stretching after golf is designed to soothe your nervous system, speed recovery, and prepare you for the next round.

Stop doing your daily stretches and you will quickly lose your hard-earned flexibility and cause your swing flaws to return.

Warming Up for Your Round

Do not ignore your warm-up. Your warm-up is designed to lubricate your joints; warm your muscles, tendons, and ligaments; activate your nervous system; and heighten your senses. All of this will produce a better round of golf.

Your body often limits your range of motion to protect a sore joint. While stretching you can actually cause your muscles to tighten up to keep a joint from being stretched too far. Using dynamic warm-up and mobilization drills will allow your joints to move much more easily because they are perceived by your brain as being less dangerous. This increased range of motion will last longer and you will be able to move more fluidly without your joints stiffening to protect themselves from injury.

When you use mobilization drills your brain is completely aware of your joints' new range of motion. This will prevent any alterations to your swing from occurring.

How to Mobilize Your Golf Muscles

For maximum results, pick the drills that hit your tightest areas and perform them at the start of your warm-up. This will give you maximum mobility, sharpen your senses, and help you have a correct, powerful, repeating golf swing. These drills will increase the range of motion in your shoulders, spine, and hips, which means you will swing with less effort and more fluidity. You will also increase you coordination and mental focus.

When you warm up before you play or practice, you are more consistent, have greater distance, and reduce swing faults.

The 29 Best Stretches for a Correct, Powerful, Repeating Golf Swing

1) Neck Rotators

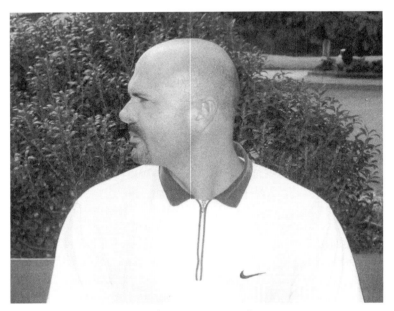

neck rotators stretch

- Stand or sit up very straight and slowly turn your head to your right side. Place your left hand on your check and face, to create a solid barrier.

- Take a deep breath in and slowly turn your head into your hand. Hold for five seconds.

- After five seconds of gentle tension, blow out your breath. Turn and look farther over your right shoulder immediately after taking pressure from your hand.

- Repeat three to five times on each side or until you no longer feel you are turning farther.

2) Neck Side Flexors

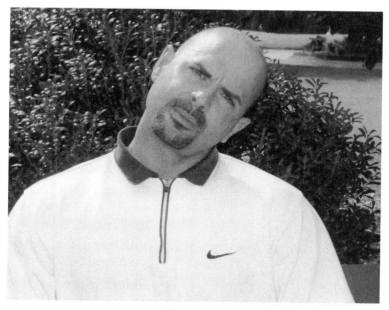

neck flexor stretch

- Sit up very straight on a chair or bench. Grab the right side of the chair or bench with your right hand. Grab the side of your head with your left hand.

- Slowly pull your neck to your left side until you feel a comfortable stretch. Take a deep breath in and bend your head into your hand without letting your head move. Hold for five seconds.

- After five seconds, exhale and gently move your head and neck to the left. Repeat three to five times on each side.

3) Upper Traps

- Stand with your left side about one foot from a wall. Reach up with your left arm.

- Look away from the wall and grab the base of your head. Lean toward the wall, let the arm holding your head

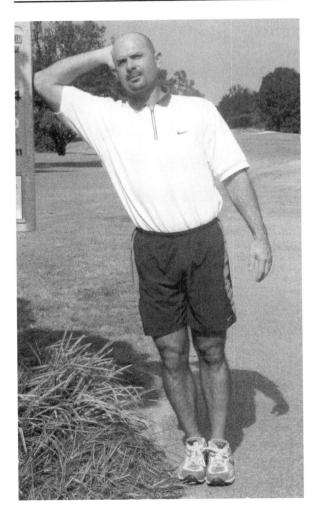

transfer the lean into your neck. Be very careful; do not apply very much force.

- When you feel a gentle stretch in your neck, take a deep breath in while you press your elbow into the wall and your head into your hands. Hold for five seconds.

- After five seconds, exhale and relax toward the wall, easily side bend your head and neck from the wall until you feel a stretch in your neck.

- Repeat three to five times on each side.

Note: If you find that one side is tighter than the other during your evaluation, stretch only your tight side. If you stretch both sides you will not restore balance to your body or swing.

upper trap stretch

4) Neck Extensors

- Stand or sit up straight and let your head drop toward your chest.

- Put your left hand on the back of your head, inhale, and push your head into your hand. Hold for five seconds.

- Relax as you let your breath out and slowly push your neck forward.

- Repeat three to five times on each side.

Note: If you feel any pain while doing this stretch, such as pain running down your neck or into your arm, stop immediately. This pain could mean that you have a cervical disc problem so you need to be checked by your doctor, physical therapist, or chiropractor.

5) Medial Shoulder Rotators and Chest

You can use a doorway or a Swiss ball to do this stretch.

Doorway stretch:

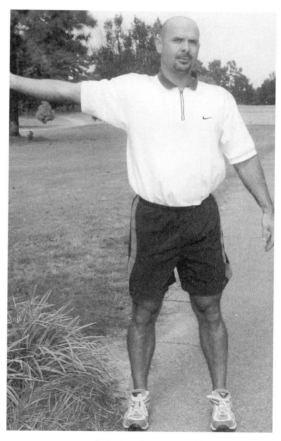

- Stand in the doorway and put your arm at a 90-degree angle (like throwing a baseball). Put your other hand and forearm up against the doorway.

- Gently turn your upper body forward around your arm (the outstretched arm), like you are pivoting around your arm.

- Once you feel a stretch in the front of your shoulder, take a deep breath and press against the doorway with your hand. Hold this position and pressure for five seconds.

- Exhale and lean forward to increase your stretch.

- Repeat three to five times on each side.

medial shoulder stretch

Note: It is very important to stop doing these stretches if you feel any discomfort in your shoulder when you perform them. If the methods bother your shoulder, check with your orthopedic doctor. Many players' shoulders are loose in the front from old injuries or poor weight-lifting technique. This stretch may be working an area that is already too loose for proper function.

6) Lateral Shoulder Rotators

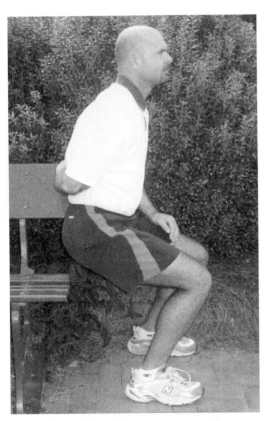

lateral shoulder rotator stretch

- Reach behind your back and grab anything that can anchor your body.
- Slowly lower yourself to the point at which you feel a stretch behind your shoulder blade.
- Take a deep breath and gently pull down on the doorknob for five seconds.
- Exhale and slide down to where you feel a slight increase in the stretch.
- Repeat three to five times on each side.

7) Rhomboids

Your rhomboids and related muscles are used to bring your shoulders toward the center line of your body.

- Kneel in front of a Swiss ball and put your elbow on the ball.
- Pull your arm across your body until it rests on the ball.
- When you feel a stretch in your upper back, inhale and try to pull your shoulder blades toward your spine.

- Hold for five seconds.
- Exhale as you release the pressure in your shoulders.
- Repeat three to five times on each side.

8) Pectoralis Major

Your chest muscles are stretched much like your medial shoulder rotators (5), except you focus on moving your arm away from the side of your body rather than rotating around your arm.

Doorway stretch:

- Stand in the doorway and put your arm at a 90-degree angle (like throwing a baseball). Put the hand and forearm of your outstretched arm up against the doorway.

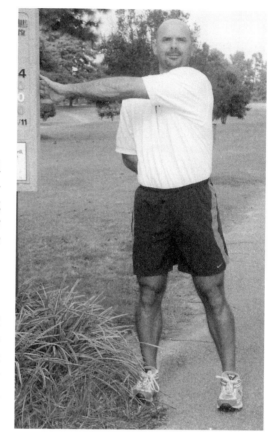

doorway stretch

- Gently lean your upper body forward into the doorway while using your hand and forearm as the point from which you stretch.

- Once you feel a stretch in your chest, take a deep breath and press against the doorway with your hand. Hold this position and pressure for five seconds.

- Exhale and lean forward to increase your stretch.

- Repeat three to five times on each side.

Swiss ball stretch:

- Place your arm over the top of the ball with your arm and shoulder at a right angle.
- Let your body drop forward as your shoulder blade moves toward your backbone.
- When you feel a stretch, inhale and press your shoulder and arm into the ball for five seconds.
- Relax and let your body drop forward while bringing your shoulder blade closer to your spine.
- Repeat three to five times on each side.

9) Wrist Extensors

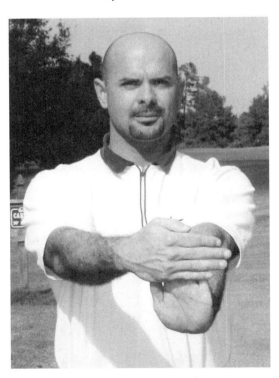

wrist extensor stretch

- Extend your left arm straight out in front of you and, reaching over or under your left arm with your right hand, grab your left hand and fingers.
- Flex your left wrist, and slightly rotate your arm toward your body to increase the stretch.
- When you feel a comfortable stretch in your wrist and fore-arm, inhale and push your left hand into your right hand for five seconds.
- Relax the pressure, exhale, and try to increase the rotation of your arm and bend in your wrist to increase the stretch of your wrist extensors.
- Repeat three to five times on each side.

10) Wrist Flexors

- Extend your left arm straight out in front of you and with your right hand push your left wrist and fingers back toward you until you feel a comfortable stretch.

- Inhale and push your fingers into your right hand and hold for five seconds.

- Release the pressure, exhale, and try to pull the wrist and fingers farther back.

- Repeat three to five times on each side.

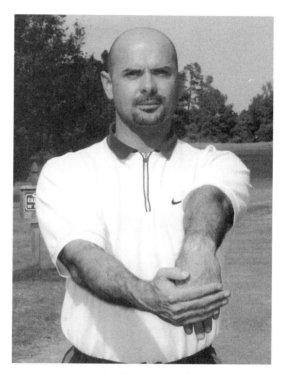

wrist flexor stretch

11) Latissimus Dorsi

- Lean against a wall with your feet about one foot from the wall and your knees slightly bent.

- Bring your hands up in front of your face like you are going to look at your palms.

- Pull your elbows into your body until they are in line with your shoulders. Pull your belly button back toward your spine as you tuck your pelvis under, and flatten your back against the wall. Make sure to keep your head and as much of your back as possible against the wall.

- Lift your hands over your head and try to touch your palms against the wall while keeping your elbows in line with your shoulders. Hold this stretch for 20 seconds.

- Perform three times.

You also perform this stretch in the opposite order:

- Lean against a wall with your feet one foot from the wall, your knees slightly bent, and a natural curve in your lower back.
- Keep your elbows in line with your shoulders and raise your hands up to the wall.
- When your hands are on the wall, pull your elbows close together, roll your pelvis backward, and flatten your spine against the wall as much as you comfortably can. Hold for 20 seconds.
- Perform three times.

12) Rectus Abdominis

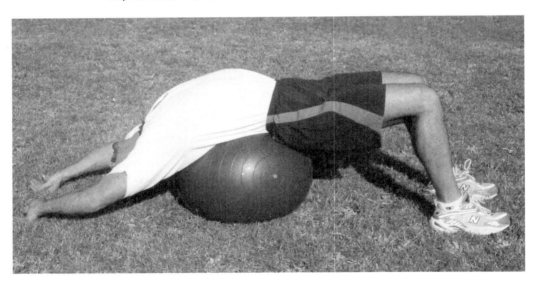

rectus abdominal stretch

The best way to stretch your stomach muscles is to lie over a Swiss ball. This not only stretches your abdominals, it also restores your ability to bend backward. Lack of ability to extend or bend your mid-back is a common link to shoulder pain and swing faults.

- Sit on the ball, walk your legs out, and roll backward until you are lying on the ball with your arms over your head.
- To increase the stretch, slowly straighten your legs, which will push your upper body farther over the ball.
- Slowly move forward and back over the ball, bringing your hands closer to the floor and then moving them away.
- Perform for at least one minute.

13) Oblique Abdominals

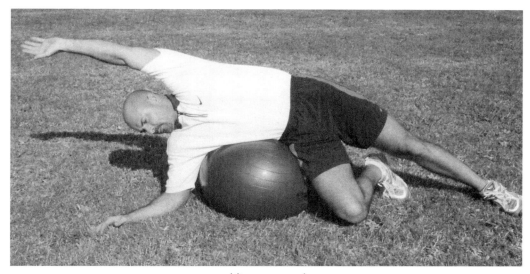

obliques stretch

- From a sitting position on a Swiss ball, roll down onto your back and then carefully roll onto your side. You may need a friend to steady the ball for you in the beginning.
- Anchor your feet against a wall.
- Grab the wrist of your top arm.
- Slowly roll forward while applying a mild tug on your upper arm. When you find a tight area, remain in that spot until your tightness relaxes.

- Gradually roll forward and back to locate tight areas, being careful not to roll off the ball. Again you may need a friend to help you or you can hold on to a stable object such as a wall or bench until you become comfortable with this stretch.
- Perform for one minute. Repeat two to three times.

14) Trunk Rotation

This stretch is very valuable to the player with a small or reduced backswing. Any limitation in your spinal rotation can reduce your golf performance.

- Lie on your back. Your hips should be flexed until your knees point to the ceiling. Be sure your lower legs relax.
- Put your left arm on your left leg, so you can help in lowering your legs or use a Swiss ball.

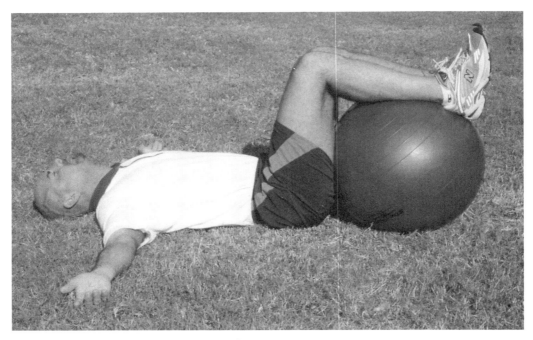

trunk rotation start

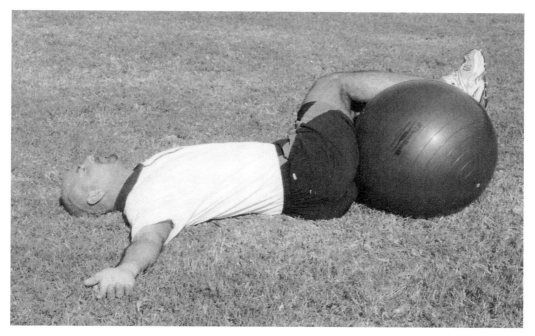

trunk rotation end

- Stretch your right arm out on the floor to hold you in place.
- Slowly let your legs roll to your left side until you feel a good stretch in your back or side.
- Hold for five seconds, then roll to your right side.
- Keep switching from your right to left sides until you can no longer go any farther or until your thighs are on the ground with your hips at a right angle.
- Perform 10 times on each side.

Note: To stretch higher up your back, bring your knees toward your chest slightly. As your hips flex, the stretch will move upward as you turn from side to side.

15) Hip Flexors

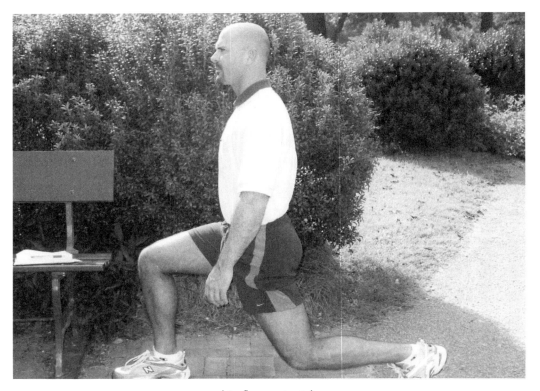

hip flexor stretch

- Get in the position of a lunge.
- Pull your belly button inward and roll your hips back to flatten your lower back.
- Move your entire pelvis forward, keeping it square to the front. If your hip flexors are very tight, your pelvis may swing out toward your rear leg.
- To deepen the stretch, reach overhead with the arm that is the same as the leg placed behind you and bend toward opposite side. You can further deepen your stretch by bending to the side toward your front leg while keeping the previous hip and arm position.

- Hold this position for 20 seconds on each side.
- Repeat on each side three times, alternating from left leg to right leg.

Note: If you determine one side is tighter than the other, you need only stretch your tight side until you have balance.

16) Lumbar Erectors

To stretch your lower back muscles, do the following:

- Lie on your back and pull both of your legs toward your chest. For the best stretch, exhale as you pull your legs to your chest.
- When you feel a nice stretch in your lower back, hold your legs with your arms and gently push your legs into your hands for five seconds. Draw your legs closer to your chest immediately after you release.
- Repeat three to five times.

Note: If you experience discomfort bringing both knees to the chest, pull one leg into your chest at a time. Repeat three to five times per leg.

17) 90/90 Hip Stretch

This may be the best stretch you can do if you have trouble clearing your hips during your swing.

- Sit on the floor with both your right and left legs bent at right angles. The left leg should be in front. The angle between your groin and legs should also form a right angle.
- Take your left hand and put it on the ground next to your left hip, with the inside of your hand facing front. This will help hold you in the correct position during the stretch.

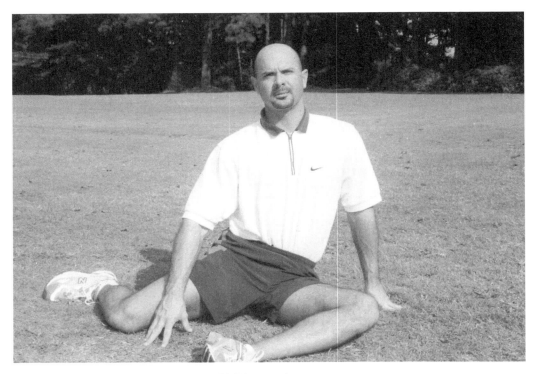

90/90 stretch start

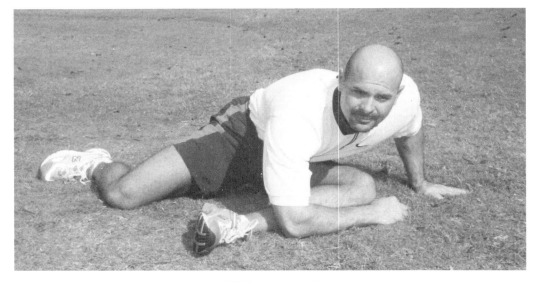

90/90 stretch end

- Lean forward from your hips. Hold this position. You should notice an increase in the curve of the small of your back.

- Inhale as you bend forward, maintaining the curve in your back and bending from your hips. To help hold the proper position, put pressure on your left hand.

- As you lean toward the floor with your upper body, make sure to bend only from your hip, keeping your chest up and your shoulders parallel to the floor; keep your eyes level to the horizon.

- When you feel a comfortable stretch in your hip socket, hold this position and press your left knee and ankle into the floor for five seconds.

- Relax, exhale, and move deeper into your stretch. Repeat three to five times per leg.

- Next, move your torso so that your head lines up with the middle of your left leg and repeat the process.

Note: As your flexibility improves you can perform the stretch with your head in line with your left foot. Perform this on each side until you reach your maximum range of movement for the day.

18) External Hip Rotators

Many programs fail to stretch your internal and external hip rotators. As a golfer, you cannot afford this oversight. Flexible hip rotators are vital to a correct, powerful, repeating golf swing.

- Stand with your feet parallel and about shoulder-width apart. Turn your left foot inward, turning from your left heel. Keep your hips square to the front.

- After you have turned your left foot inward as far as you can, hold your foot pressed into the ground with your left knee slightly bent but held stiff to brace yourself.

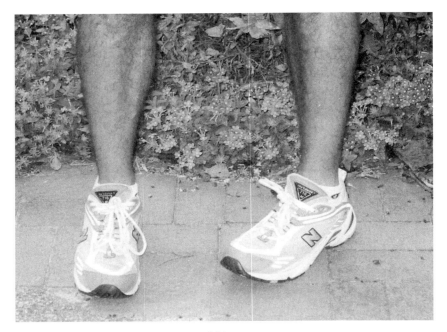

external hip rotators

- Turn your hips to the left without moving your left foot.
- When you feel a comfortable stretch in your left hip, hold your pelvis in that position, take a breath in, and try to turn your left foot back to your left, like trying to return to the starting position. Do not let your foot or leg move; you are just trying to stimulate your pelvic muscles. Hold for five seconds.
- Exhale as you relax the stretch and move your pelvis further into a new stretch position.
- Repeat three to five times per side.

19) Internal Hip Rotators

- Start in the same position as the External Hip Rotator stretch.
- Turn your left foot outward as far as possible, turning from your heel.

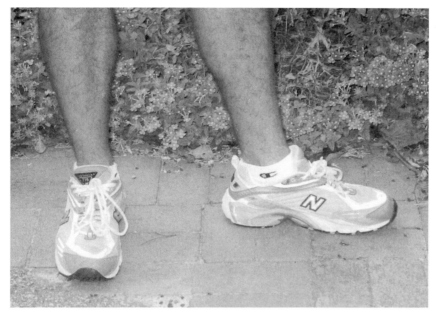

internal hip rotators

- Hold your left leg still and turn your hips toward your right side.
- When you feel a nice stretch in your hip, inhale. Keep your left knee stiff and leg steady as you try to turn your left leg against the ground.
- Exhale and move your hips to the right until you feel a deeper stretch.
- Repeat three to five times per leg.

20) Groin Stretch

This is a traditional groin stretch used by many players.

- Sit on the floor with a straight posture and with your feet together and your heels pulled toward your groin as far as you can. Your forearms should be resting on your shins and your hands holding on to your ankles.

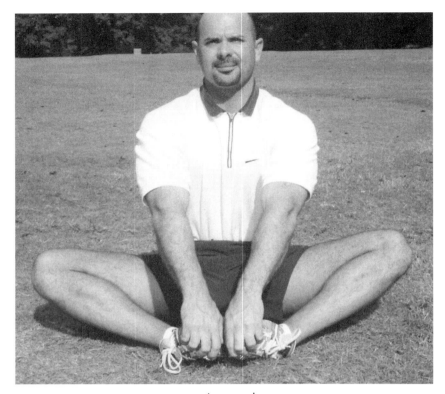

groin stretch

- Take a deep breath in, as you slightly press on your legs to the point of a comfortable stretch.
- Push up against your arms with your upper legs for five seconds.
- Exhale, relax the pressure, and gently push down with your arms to deepen the stretch.
- Repeat three to five times.

21) Rocking Groin Stretch

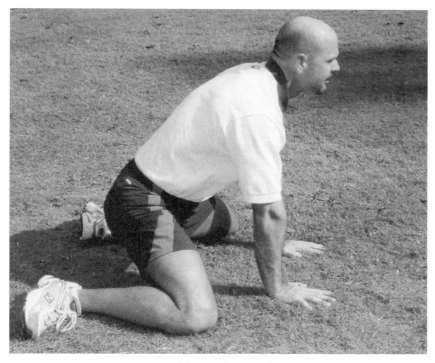

rocking groin stretch

Perform this on thick carpet, a mat, or grass to cushion your knees.

- Kneel on the floor and spread your knees as far apart as you can comfortably. Place your hands on the ground in front of you.
- Rock forward until you feel a comfortable stretch in your upper groin.
- Inhale and gently squeeze your knees into the floor for five seconds.
- Exhale and relax your groin as you sink into a deeper stretch.
- Perform for three to five repetitions.

Note: You should perform this stretch from a variety of angles, with your upper body upright, slightly leaning forward and parallel to the ground. You can also improve the stretch by slightly rolling your hips to the left and right once in the stretch position. It is very important to stretch your groin and upper thigh when they are tight or it will be nearly impossible to keep a stable swing axis. A tight groin can inhibit your ability to clear your hips during your swing.

22) Standing Hamstring Stretch

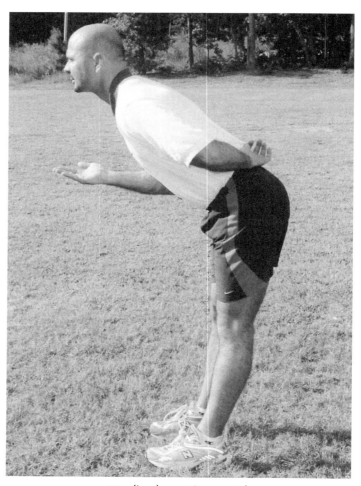

standing hamstring stretch

- Stand with your feet close together and parallel to each other. Keep your legs straight and stick your buttocks out until you have an arch in your lower back.

- Bend forward at your waist, without rounding your back, until you feel a comfortable stretch in your hamstrings. You may feel the stretch behind your knee or underneath your buttocks, depending on where you are tightest.

- Hold this position for 20 seconds.

- Relax, stand straight up for one to two seconds, and repeat the stretch.

- Repeat three to five times or until you do not feel your hamstrings getting looser.

23) Lying Hamstring Stretch

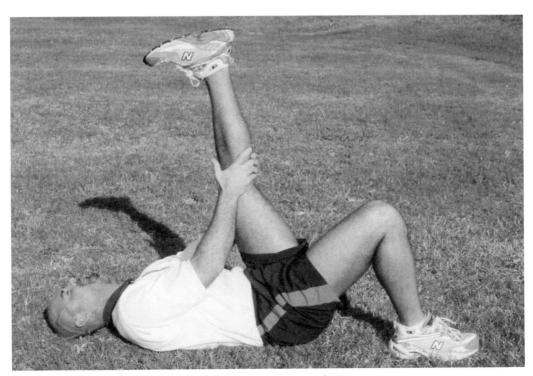

lying hamstring stretch

You will feel this stretch mostly behind your knee.

- Lie on your back.
- Bend your left leg and with your hands, grab the knee of your bent leg and lift it up until your thigh is at a right angle to the floor.
- Flex your toes back toward your knee as far as you can and then slowly straighten your leg without letting your left thigh move in your hands.
- When you reach the point of a comfortable stretch, hold for 20 seconds and then switch sides.
- Repeat three to five times per leg.

24) Supine Quadriceps Stretch

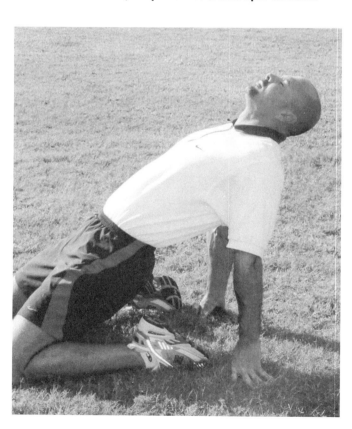

- Kneel on a mat, thick carpet, or grass to protect your knees. Place your hands behind you.
- Pull your belly button in and tuck your pelvis under.
- Hold a comfortable stretch in the upper portion of your thigh for 20 seconds.
- Repeat three to five times or until you no longer feel the stretch deepen.

supine quadricep stretch

25) Swiss Ball Quadriceps Stretch

You will feel this stretch around your knee.

- Begin in a crouched position with your left foot and ankle on the ball. For more control and stability, put your left hand next to your left foot. If you have trouble getting into this stretch try using a smaller ball.

- From this upright position, pull your belly button in and tuck your buttocks under to flatten your back. This will increase your stretch.

- To deepen the stretch, keep pushing your hip forward.

- Press your foot into the ball for five seconds. Relax for five seconds and increase the stretch.

- Repeat three to five times on each side.

26) Calf Stretch

To stretch the big bulky portion of your calf, do the following:

- Stand on the edges of a step, curb, or a block and let your left heel drop toward the floor while keeping your leg straight.

- Hold for 20 seconds and switch to your right leg.

- Repeat three to five times per leg.

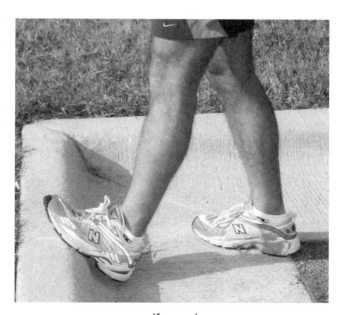

calf stretch

To stretch the long slender muscle of your calf, do the following:

- Bend your knee forward at the bottom of the previous stretch. You will feel the stretch move down your calf toward your heel. Do not let the stretch move into your heel.
- Hold the stretch for 20 seconds.
- Switch from right to left three to five times.

27) Press-up

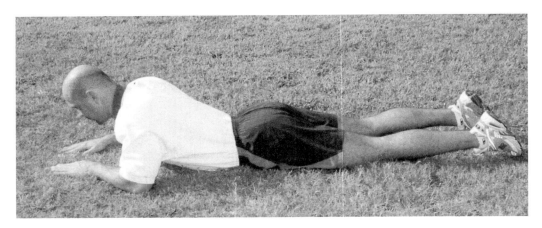

press-up

- Lie on your stomach with your hands just outside the top of your shoulders.
- Inhale deeply and begin to press up your upper body, like starting a push-up but keep your hips on the floor. As you push up, exhale to help bend your back. Make sure to relax your back and buttock muscles.
- Hold your top position until you need to take a breath.
- Inhale as you slowly lower your body to the floor.
- Repeat 10 times.

Note: This is not a strength drill but a mobilization exercise to help you return normal range of motion to your lower spine. It is not unusual to feel some discomfort during the first three to five lifts, but it should gradually decrease between the fifth and tenth stretch. If you have discomfort with every one, you may need to consult with your doctor.

28) Foam Roller Mobilizations

Note: If you have restrictions in the Push-up and/or Torso Turn tests, it is important to have a doctor check for arthritis of your spine. Before trying the Press-up and Foam Roller and Longitudinal Mobilizations stretches (27, 28, and 29) get it checked. If you have arthritis in your spine some of your vertebrae may be fused together. If you perform these drills as a means to reach normal range of motion with this condition, you may fracture your spine. Get medical clearance to do these drills.

- Place a three- to four-inch foam roller perpendicular to your spine just below your shoulder blades.
- Hold your neck in your hands, making sure not to hold your head or you may experience neck discomfort during the drill.
- Exhale as you allow yourself to drop backward over the roller toward the floor. There may be some discomfort so go slowly and only as far back as you can comfortably.
- Hold the end position for three to five seconds. Each vertebra should be mobilized three to five times.

Note: You should do this drill before golf or exercise, or during the middle of the day and in the evening; twice a day is enough to improve your spinal flexibility. If you feel any discomfort in your spine after the drills, you are probably doing too much. Reduce your repetitions. If you still feel pain, consult your doctor.

29) Longitudinal Mobilizations

Note: It is often helpful to perform this stretch, in which you lay on the roller lengthwise, at the middle or end of your day. This lets gravity stretch the ligaments in front of the spine, which helps return the optimal curvature to your spine. The better your alignment, the better your turn during your golf swing.

- Place the roller along your spine from the base of your head to your tailbone. Your knees should be bent and your feet should be flat on the floor.
- To improve the rotational mobility of your spine, let your hips and shoulders roll in opposite directions on the roller. Repeat until you feel loose.
- Start with five minutes a day and work up to fifteen minutes per day.

How to Cure the 28 Most Common Swing Flaws

The following is a table of the 28 most common swing flaws and the stretches you should include in your daily program to solve your most common swing fault.

Here's how it works: Let's say your most common swing fault is taking the clubface back closed. You would look on the left side of the page until you find fault number 8: Taking the clubface back closed. On the right side directly across from fault number 8 are the stretches you will perform to help correct this flaw. These include:

- Neck Rotators. Both sides. (1)
- Medial Shoulder Rotators and Chest. The "r" means you will only stretch your right side. (5r)
- Lateral Shoulder Rotators. The "l" means you will only stretch your left side. (6l)
- Rhomboids. The "l" means you will only stretch your left side. (7l)

Swing Faults and Fixes

Swing Fault	Fix
1. Poor posture at address	2–5, 15, 22, 26, 28
2. Losing your grip during the swing	1–10
3. Misalignment of clubface at address	1–10, 13–15
4. Misalignment of body at address	1–29
5. Stance too wide	17, 18, 22
6. Tension at address	1–29
7. Clubhead moves inside too quickly	1, 3, 7, 8, 10, 11, 13, 14
8. Taking the clubface back closed	1, 5 (right side), 6 (left side), 7 (left side)
9. Flat laid off backswing	11, 12
10. Body turn completed too early	17–21, 24, 25
11. Incomplete body turn	11–16
12. Overswing (bending left arm)	3, 5r, 6l, 7l, 17–21, 24, 25
13. Wrong plane (too upright or too flat)	1, 3, 5, 6, 7, 8, 10–21, 24, 25
14. Club jammed behind body	6r, 7r, 11r, 13, 14, 17l, 18l
15. Poor weight transfer, no legs	15, 17–22, 24, 25
16. Early release, casting the clubhead	17–21, 24, 25
17. Poor body release (dominant left side)	11–21, 24, 25
18. No extension past impact	11–15, 17–19, 20r, 25r
19. Poor follow-through position	11–15, 17–19, 20r, 25r
20. Excessive head movement	1–6, 17–21, 24, 25
21. Slices and pulls	3, 5, 6, 17–21, 24, 25
22. Hooking and pushing	3, 5r, 7r, 10r, 11r, 17–21, 24, 25
23. The Shank	1–29
24. Topped-skulled fat shots	1–29
25. Putting (excessive body motion/ poor spine axis)	17–21, 24, 25
26. Poor power development (for women only)	3, 14–16
27. Loss of mobility (for seniors only)	1–29
28. Loss of power (for seniors only)	1–29

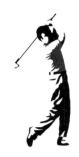

CHAPTER FOUR

Golf Strong:
Strength Training for Golf

Golf is a dynamic sport that requires powerful, repeated muscle contractions. That's why golf conditioning must include strength training instead of static, isometric training.

The shortening and lengthening of the muscle fibers during training is important because golf requires these muscle contractions in every swing and body movement. Typically, golfers use eccentric contractions to decelerate and control or stabilize the body; for example, eccentric contractions occur in your thigh muscles as you finish your follow-through. Concentric contractions occur in the front of your shoulder as you accelerate the club downward to hit the ball.

You can perform isotonic exercise with body weight; free weights, such as dumbbells or barbells; medicine balls; rubber tubing; and weight machines. Although there is no one best form of isotonic exercise for the golfer, each form has its advantages and disadvantages; for example, body weight is always available, but you cannot easily change your body weight as you get stronger to provide greater resistance.

Using free weights is a cost-effective form of training that requires great control during lifting because there is no guide path or movement track such as that provided by a weight machine. Using free weights forces you to stabilize the weight in all directions while moving it in the primary movement pattern. This works secondary muscle groups that stabilize the joints you are exercising, but requires greater skill and supervision due to less control of the path the weight travels. One additional benefit of many weight machines is their ability to vary the resistance during the exercise range of motion.

Another type of resistance golfers commonly use is rubber tubing or rubber cords. This form of resistance is desirable because it is cost-effective, easy to travel with, and potent—the farther you stretch the cord, the greater the resistance you generate.

Whatever type of isotonic exercise you do, the important factor is movement. The joints move and the muscles lengthen and shorten, mimicking the actions you do when driving, chipping, or putting. Most exercises in this chapter are isotonic. They use free weights, rubber tubing, and weight machines to provide you with a resistance program using whatever methods are available to you.

Isokentic resistance training uses a constant velocity and changing amounts of resistance. It uses a highly technical and expensive machine that does not allow most players to use this form of resistance in their training. Isokentic machines are used extensively in rehabilitating injuries and in research, and they have given sports scientists important information regarding the strengths and weaknesses of the muscular system of the golfer.

Within each type of resistance for increasing strength there are two primary forms of exercise: single joint and multiple joint. In a single-joint exercise the golfer is working one primary joint and muscle group; for example, a knee-extension exercise involves movement only at the knee joint and primarily works the quadriceps (front of thigh) muscle. A multiple-joint exercise is one that works many muscles and muscle groups, and includes movement at several joints simultaneously. A squat is a multiple-joint exercise that works the gluteals, quadriceps, hamstrings, calf muscles, and others, with movement occurring at the hip, knee, and ankle joints.

Both types of exercise are beneficial to the golfer. Multiple-joint exercises work more muscles and joints simultaneously and certainly are time efficient. Multiple-joint exercises require great balance. Proper form and training are essential to achieving the optimum benefit and preventing injury. Single-joint exercises are beneficial when one muscle group is weak and the player has a muscle imbalance requiring exercise for one muscle group.

Power Training for Golf

Training the muscular system for power involves intense, explosive contractions that are performed rapidly, because power is speed applied to strength. Because of the increased risk of injury, we do not advocate using traditional exercise patterns with weight machines and free weights and simply performing them with fast, uncontrolled movements. Instead, players should use special types of resistance training to improve power in golf.

One primary type of resistance training for power in golf is plyometrics. Plyometrics were initially used as a method for improving explosive power in Eastern Europe and now have become a popular training method throughout the world. Plyometrics condition the body through dynamic resistance training that follows a specific pattern.

Plyometric exercises begin with a rapid stretching of the muscle using an eccentric or shortening muscle contraction. This is immediately followed by an explosive shortening of the muscle. A classic example of a plyometric exercise would be a box jump. An athlete stands on a wooden or metal box about 18 inches high, jumps off the box, and upon contact with the ground, reverses his or her direction to jump into the air as high as possible. The quicker a player changes direction the more explosive or intense the plyometric program is.

The goal of plyometric training is to train the muscles and nervous system to quickly stretch the muscles by shortening the muscles at maximal force and speed. Plyometrics have been used for many years to induce explosive strength and power in sprinters and other athletes.

The golf swing itself is a plyometric exercise. As you make your backswing, the abdominal muscles are stretched on your lead side. As your shoulder, arm, and torso explosively rotate forward to contact the ball, your abdominals are shortening, as in a plyometric exercise. The eccentric contraction pre-stretches the muscle and surrounding tissues; enables an explosive, concentric contraction; and provides a training stimulus to increase strength.

Power training for golf uses these plyometric movements. Athletes use specific drills for the lower body and medicine balls for the upper body and trunk. You can safely perform explosive movement patterns using medicine balls, which allow you to train with plyometrics in an exciting, golf-specific way.

Resistance Training Adaptations

We can break down adaptations to resistance training into two forms: nervous system and muscular development. Improvements involving the nervous system can occur in as little as two weeks after starting a resistance-training program. When you begin to lift weights, and feel stronger after a week or two, this is primarily because the nervous system becomes more efficient in how it recruits or talks to the muscle. This, in turn, makes you feel stronger, even though little change has occurred within the muscle itself.

The second type of adaptation to strength training involves muscular adaptation. Scientists still debate the exact mechanism of this adaptation. No matter how it works, scientists agree that it takes six weeks of training for muscular adaptation to occur. Strength-training programs lasting six to twenty-four weeks will increase the percentage of lean body mass and result in a lower percentage of body fat.

One common myth about lifting weights for golf is that it will make a player bulky and muscle bound, and will have a negative effect on the golf swing. This could happen but only if you do not follow a strength-training program specific to golfers. A golf-specific training program does not involve heavy, maximal-effort lifts but instead light to moderate resistance levels with high repetitions that build strength and muscular endurance, not bulk and size.

Another myth associated with resistance training is that it will cause stiffness and loss of flexibility. Again, a program specifically for a golfer, with a total conditioning program including flexibility, will prevent flexibility loss, optimize performance, and prevent injury.

Designing a Strength-Training Program

Developing a needs analysis is the first step in designing a strength-training program for any athlete. The concept of specificity is vitally important when designing your training program. Every resistance exercise must address the demands of the activity and consider the biomechanical requirements of the sport. Biomechanical analysis helps sports scientists tailor training programs for golfers.

Much of my program evolved from the continued research at the Centinela Hospital Biomechanics Laboratory. Since 1983 they have been testing professional golfers to evaluate their golf swings. They study the minute details of the golf swing by gathering data using high-speed cameras, electromyography, and computers. From these studies, they isolated the muscles most prominent at impact in the backswing and the downswing and in the follow-through.

The following findings were most helpful:

1. A good golf swing uses the left side of the body as much as the right. A good golf swing is a balanced activity; the net output on the right and left side muscles are equal. Many instructors and golfers still emphasize the left side in the belief that it gives the power for the right-hand golfer. Their studies of the hips and shoulders show that the right side is at least as active as the left. The exercises I recommend give equal emphasis to both sides of the body.

2. The hips initiate movement into the ball. It is clear from the data that the hip muscles become active before the upper body turns into the shot. Each specific muscle of the hip has a unique job. Each fires in a precise sequence to initiate the motion of the golf swing.

3. The body acts like a whip during the golf swing. The power of the golf swing comes from the synchronous coordination of precise muscle firing throughout the swing. The body acts like a whip. The feet push against the ground causing a ground-reaction force that travels through the hips, the trunk, and, finally, out the arms. The arms and trunk play a small role in adding "power" to the swing but are an important part of the sequence. If the sequence of the swing is disturbed at any point in the swing, the momentum and power dissipate throughout the body. The only choice the body has is to substitute and try again to initiate the "power" after the point of disruption. This puts the golfer at risk of injury.

4. Trunk rotation and flexibility are especially important. The biggest difference noted between pros and amateurs was in the trunk rotation. Older and less skilled players used less than half the trunk rotation of younger or more skilled players. The lack of flexibility and strength explains why ability decreases with age. Golfers gradually lose the arc motion that enables the body to transmit maximum velocity to the club at impact. Inadequate use of the trunk muscles caused a compensation for the lack of sufficient rotation to attain optimal clubbed speed at impact. "Muscling" the ball resulted in a swing that was too fast and placed added stress on the muscles and joints. As the rounds progress, the muscles become increasingly prone to fatigue and injury.

    These findings indicate the benefits of increased flexibility and conditioned muscles, tendons, and ligaments.

5. The scapular muscles and rotator-cuff muscles are crucial in the golf swing. Many golf-related shoulder injuries can be traced to problems in these two groups of muscles. These muscles help to precisely position the upper extremity and hence prevent injury. The rotator-cuff muscles are very active in the swing and are vulnerable to overuse and microtramua. The scapular muscles stabilize the scapula, which allows the arms to function properly.

   This indicates the need for a rotator-cuff and scapular-muscle conditioning program.

6. The research showed that skilled golfers more efficiently use their muscles, such as when swinging the club. The pros used a lower percentage of their maximum muscular output potential as they swung the club compared to the amateurs tested.

   This indicates the need for good golf swing instruction and practice.

7. The data shows that men and women utilize the same muscle-firing patterns. The timing and intensity relative to the overall strength of the muscle firing is the same. This information reveals that the instructional techniques and exercise programs can be the same for men and women.

The conclusion from this information is that any exercise program designed for golfers should emphasize both sides of the body, focus on the hips as they start the swing, develop trunk rotation and increase flexibility, condition the scapular muscles and rotator cuff to protect them from injury, condition all the muscles of the body to protect it from the whiplike motion of the golf swing, feature good golf instruction to develop an efficient swing. The program is equally applicable to men and women.

Components of a Strength-Training Program

In designing a training regimen for golf, consider the following components:

- **Sets—groupings of repetitions within a resistance training program:** Typically multiple sets of an exercise are required to improve strength and muscular endurance. For golf, we recommend two to four sets.

- **Repetitions—the number of repetitions you perform per set:** This determines the amount of work and regulates the exercise intensity. Exercise sets with three to six repetitions normally develop power and strength when you use higher resistance loads. Sets of 10 to 15 repetitions develop muscular strength, as well as local muscle endurance due to the higher number of repetitions per set. Sets with 20 to 25 repetitions help train for endurance and are geared for athletes such as marathon runners. What is the optimal number of repetitions for a golfer? Most experts recommend sets ranging from 10 to 15 repetitions. This number provides strength-training stimulus as well as endurance, both of which are needed for golf.

- **Intensity—how much weight you lift:** The exercise intensity is set using the repetition maximum, or RM, system. This involves selecting an appropriate weight for an exercise set so that all desired repetitions can be performed without breaking proper form, and so you feel significant muscle fatigue during the last one or two repetitions of that set; for example, choosing a two-pound weight to do bicep curls for ten repetitions would probably not cause fatigue by the ninth or tenth repetition. To properly apply the repetition maximum system takes some trial and error when beginning a strength-training program because the goal is specific: to choose a weight or resistance at which you can perform the preset number of repetitions without breaking form and yet fatigue the muscle.

Since a higher number of repetitions in a set are rec-ommended for golfers, the relative amount of weight used is going to be lower because you must be able to do many repetitions with that weight.

- **Movement cadence—speed:** The speed that you move the weight has a tremendous effect on workout quality. It is important that you emphasize a slow, controlled movement when you work on weight machines, free weights, and rubber tubing. This will ensure that you are raising and lowering or pushing and pulling the weight, which means you will be working the muscle in both the shortening (concentric) and lengthening (eccentric) phase, similar to what happens when playing golf.

- **Frequency—how often you do sessions:** Most strength-training programs recommend rest between sessions of exercise. Depending on what other elements a player is emphasizing in the total conditioning program, the train-ing frequency can range from one time per week to three to four times per week. Most strength-training programs recommend three times per week to build strength, with a day of rest between training sessions. Some players may lift weights every day, but they alternate what muscle groups and body areas they work to allow a day of recovery for the worked muscle groups.

- **Rest—time between sets:** One factor closely tied to a golf training program is rest. A swing lasts about two seconds followed by about a minute of rest. During practice, this rest period is reduced to about ten seconds. Therefore, a golfer's program should emphasize various rest peri-ods of approximately 25 to 30 seconds when working on endurance and 60 to 90 seconds when working on strength and power. This work/rest cycle provides stress to the muscles similar to that experienced when playing and practicing golf, and it metabolically stresses the sys-tems that provide energy to the working muscles as if you were playing.

Strength-Training Workouts

With the essential design elements in mind, let's look at putting them into workouts. Be aware of these three points:

- Do not lift weights immediately before you play golf. You don't want to be fatigued while you perform skilled motor tasks like putting. It is better to do strength training on days when golf workouts are lighter. You can lift weights after playing golf.

- Don't apply the status quo with strength training. Every good program must be updated following the principle of overload. If you always use a two-pound weight when doing ten repetitions, this will, in time, become too easy. To avoid training at an intensity level that is too low, add resistance when you no longer fatigue at the end of an exercise set. Some players increase the number of repetitions by three to five with the same weight; when that becomes easy, they return to the original number of repetitions per set but with a heavier weight.

- Avoid compensation. If you use too much weight, you will use bigger muscle groups and improper movement patterns that might produce injuries. Stay within your limits of resistance, not your friends' or opponents' levels.

Creating a Home Gym

If your impression of the public gym is that of a crowded and far away fitness factory, you might be one of the increasing number of people who are opting to bypass the crowds and stay fit by setting up a home gym. The home exercise industry is booming. Americans spend about $1.7 billion on equipment every year, and it's easy to understand why. You can't beat the commute to your living room, and you can workout at 3 A.M. on Sunday if you really want to. You don't have to pay membership fees, wait in line for the shower or deal with any unidentified biological matter that doesn't contain your own DNA.

Yet, despite all the convenience, home exercisers have a high drop out rate. This article will show you how to avoid this problem and the accompanying guilt by sharing how to plan your home gym carefully.

Locate the Right Exercise Space

Wherever you decide to place your home gym, it should be a comfortable and inviting area. You can create a superb gym regardless of whether it is located in a small studio apartment, townhouse, condominium, home office, or an estate. But, if its cramped, dim, drab, dingy, or stuffy, this isn't a place you're going to want to spend time. If it's bright, organized, uncluttered, fresh and attractive, it's a lot easier to get excited about exercising.

Natural light from windows and skylights works best to motivate exercise spirit, and windows and skylights can provide a visual distraction. Walls and mirrors can take you only so far. If the space you have chosen is dark, or you work out at night, provide enough artificial lighting so that you're not lulled into thinking you're at a romantic dinner or chained in a dungeon.

Make sure you have an option for fresh air ventilation, if possible. As a minimum, heating a cooling system or portable fans should provide air circulation. You'll appreciate the right lighting and refreshing air in all seasons. Remember, you're here to breathe deeply and work out, and you need a gym environment that proves irresistible.

Hardwood floors are an ideal surface on which to place equipment. They are stable and easy to clean. Their downside is that they scratch easily and are noisier. This is especially important to consider if you have family members or neighbors that don't appreciate your early or late night exercise sessions. To protect your floors and ease the noise concern, rubber mats are available and specially designed to fit under exercise equipment or cover an entire area. If you use carpeting or a rug, a short pile indoor-outdoor cut is the best. It should be a commercial (heavy-duty) quality and have little or no padding underneath. Equipment can leave an almost permanent imprint on thickly padded surfaces, which can create a less stable exercising surface. If you exercise on the floor, use an exercise mat to protect the carpeting from sweat and cushion your body. Choose carpet color combinations that will not show dirt, machinery oil, or foot traffic patterns.

Mirrors not only help you check your exercise form and posture, but if placed correctly, can turn a small area into a seemingly larger space. Mirrors can help create a feeling of openness and a sense of spaciousness when it does not physically exist. A four-by-six to eight-foot mirror placed horizontally on a wall about 18 inches from the floor can totally recreate the atmosphere of any exercise area.

Finally, it's nice to consider the positive aspect or distraction of watching TV and listening to music while exercising. You can use your cordless phone, too. The obvious attraction for many is distraction and the fact that you can accomplish at least two or three tasks simultaneously in a time slot designated for your exercise. For example, you can get your exercise in, call a couple of friends, and keep an ear turned to your favorite TV show. To the purist this may seem like a cop out, but if time is at a premium, it helps you pass the time, you're seeing the results you want, and it keeps exercising FUN-do it.

Home Equipment Purchases

Here's a primer on how to go about selecting your home gym equipment. Before you look at the Home Gym Pre-Assessment Questionnaire (page 92) and the Checklist for Home Equipment Purchases (page 94), plant the following thought firmly in your mind: regardless of how big or small your home gym is, whether you have an entire room or a corner spot dedicated, try to minimize the necessity of taking down and setting up equipment.

Let me state it more strongly. Forget it! It doesn't work! More programs and good intentions fall short because of a failure to commit space to allow for permanent setup of equipment. Having to set up and take down equipment gives you another excuse for not exercising. If space is at a premium in your home, realize that you don't need a lot of this precious commodity to set up a gym. If you shop smart, you can buy equipment that fits into small spaces nicely, is versatile enough to offer more than one type of exercise, and won't compromise the effectiveness and safety of your workout.

Aerobic Equipment

The simplest and least expensive cardiovascular equipment is a good pair of walking, running, or cross-training shoes. Regardless of how you strengthen your heart, you'll probably need at least a couple of pairs of good shoes to complement the cardio activity you participate in. Different activities often require different shoes, and your shoes need time to air out before the next workout. So, it's a good idea to visit a high end specialty shoe store if you don't know the types of shoes you need for your workouts.

Some examples of the more popular cardiovascular equipment you have to choose from are treadmills, steppers/climbers, elliptical trainers, ski machines, lateral trainers (side-to-side pushing or sliding movement), recumbent bikes, and rowing machines. Note that the stationary cycle or spin-training craze warrants that you try the new breed of high performance "spin" training bikes. This newer breed of spin-training bike is more fully adjustable to your body's dimensions, but try before you buy! Stationary bikes have come a long way.

Many safety features, different types of electronics, and optional upgrade choices are available on this huge selection of choices. Your choice really comes down to a personal decision (what do you love to do?) and variety.

Remember the truism "know thyself." Find several activities you really enjoy and purchase a couple of pieces of equipment so you can cross-train indoors when necessary. Probably the most solid choice you can make is to purchase a fully automated treadmill. If you despise walking or running on treadmills, forget this recommendation! Complement this choice with a manual resistance bike, climber/stepper, or rowing machine. Cross-training between aerobic exercises will keep you from getting bored out of your head and provide new physiological stimulation. You can even create a sport conditioning circuit. This type of approach will keep you enthusiastic about exercise and keep you from hitting exercise plateaus and falling into an exercise rut. Remember, you can exercise outdoors, too!

Strength Equipment

Don't believe it when you read, or someone tells you, that weight machines or multistation gyms are the safest. Safest compared to what? It is true you can't drop a weight on the floor, or your toe, when using these units. But, what good is this safety feature if you end up wrecking your shoulder because an exercise motion is incorrectly designed and you have no way to correct it, or you get into and out of a machine incorrectly and tear off your upper limbs? On the other hand, like most pieces of exercise equipment, machines aren't necessarily bad if they're used properly and designed correctly.

The previous paragraph illustrates how unfounded biases sometimes blind you to the big picture and can lead you astray, get you hurt, prevent you from getting the results you want, and keep you lost in the hardware jungle. Read on so you can get the whole story.

A wide variety of strength exercise equipment is available for you to train your entire body effectively. There is overlap from category to category. Strength exercise equipment includes the following:

Freeweights (Dumbbells, barbells and hand-held weights can be used to create a myriad of exercise options that are biomechanically correct.)

Multistation weight machines. (They have their pros and cons and are generally pulley/cable systems that are routed to selectorized plates or weight stacks, although some movement are limited by what cable connects to, for example, a straight bar or chest flye attachment.)

Pulley/cable systems. (As mentioned, multistation gyms are often pulley/cable systems that use weight stacks for resistance and the cable connects to various exercise devices.)

Elastic resistance cable or tubing. (Elastic resistance can be classified as a cable system and can be used without pulleys or directed through pulleys. It can be attached to the wall or a door frame and provides unlimited and versatile exercise options. This stuff really works if you get pieces of tubing that are strong enough to effectively resist the exercise movement!)

Training without equipment. (Calisthenics and your own body weight have limitations with regard to progressive overload and working out at the right level of resistance.)

Choose strength equipment that offers you the option to increase resistance as you get stronger. Free weights, multistation weight machines, pulley/cable systems, and elastic tubing are examples of equipment that can provide progressive overload. This type of equipment allows you to increase weight once you can perform more repetitions than your recommended range. This keeps you progressing and keeps the results coming.

Free Weights

Barbells and dumbbells generally have free weights or weight plates attached to them. Barbells are long, straight bars that allow you to attach weight plates on each end of the bar. When loaded, you need two hands to lift them. Dumbbells are short bars with weight plates on both ends. Usually you lift one with each hand or use a single dumbbell in both hands, depending on the exercise. The plates can be attached securely with retaining collars or more permanent fixtures that eliminate the possibility of the free weight falling off during exercise.

Free weights are great because they don't take up much room, are inexpensive and versatile compared to machines, and offer numerous exercises that are biomechanically correct. You don't need $100,000 worth of equipment to get a great strength workout, yet you can replicate $100,000 worth of exercises with them!

Free weights work with your body, not against it, if you've been instructed correctly with regard to technique and you're using the right exercises. Free weights require balance, stabilization, and coordination. That's important because what you do in everyday life, and the sports you participate in, also require balance, stabilization, and coordination.

Free weight workouts don't take much time if you avoid adjustable dumbbells that require you to slide weight plates on and off and then secure them with safety collars so they don't slide off onto your pretty face. Instead, go for fixed dumbbells. These are not adjustable and are very durable with minimal maintenance. They don't come apart on you. You grab the pair you need, do your exercise, and you're on to the next one.

One very effective system I have seen on the market, with regard to cost and space efficiency, is the PowerBlock dumbbell system. The PowerBlock gives you a whole set of dumbbells in your home at minimal cost, and its unique design doesn't require much space. It's nice to have the versatility without taking up the space of an entire wall, which is required of a dumbbell rack that houses 10 to 15 pairs of dumbbells. Three sets are available which go up to 45, 90 and 120 pounds, and you can change from 5 pounds to 120 pounds in seconds.

When using free weights:

- Keep your concentration and focus

- Lift a weight that you can control.

- If the weight is hard to balance or control because it's

too heavy or you've reached a point of fatigue, lower the weight and start again with less weight.

- Remove the weight carefully from the rack and replace it with precision and control back onto its stand. Many injuries during strength training come from carelessly picking up or returning weight to storage racks, or the floor!

- Learn how to move into and out of an exercise safely.

Multistation Weight Machines

Many home multistation strength gyms require you to push, pull, or curl in a predetermined range. Some companies like Tuff Stuff, are now making commercial quality equipment that allows the user to define the range of motion. This trickling down to home gym designs that allow greater biomechanical adjustability to some degree. You've probably experienced a machine that doesn't feel right or creates discomfort in a joint. You could be performing an ineffective or unsafe exercise with no option to modify it. Before you buy, try out the machine and each exercise it offers. The range of motion should feel natural and comfortable, and at no point during the movement should you feel discomfort or pain. Additionally, many multistation gyms do not have many exercise options. Make sure you target all your major muscle groups. Don't trust that all manufacturers know what they're doing and have your best interest placed first with regard to exercise design and selection. Often, they don't.

If you choose to purchase a higher end home gym, you'll find it has multiple weight stacks, has a removable bench that lies flat and inclines at several different angles, and it can train most, if not all of the major muscle groups. Plus, you can push yourself without needing a partner to spot you since the weight can't fall on you and it can take up as little as four by eight feet in space. Check to make sure your ceiling height accommodates the machine. Multiple weight stacks require fewer adjustments and cable connections as you move from exercise to exercise, and more than one person can work out at a time. The guide rods and cables will operate smoothly and quietly.

Helpful Hint: Adding a full range of dumbbells to your workout
arsenal will add all the strength exercise options you'll ever
need, and you can use the bench that comes with the multistation gym.

Weight machines usually come with a stack of weights,
although there are other effective options. Like composite rods
or rubber resistance bands. When using stacked plates or selectorized plates, you select the amount of weight you want by
inserting a T-shaped pin through a small hole drilled in each
weight plate.

As I have discussed, one problem with machines is that
they're usually designed as "one size fits all." You've heard that
promise before and you know what it gets you. The low end
multistation gyms available at discount stores or sporting good
stores tend to have this problem. Most machines use a cam
design to alter the amount of weight you work against at different points throughout the range of motion. This represents a
strength curve and what is called variable resistance. Do you
think your strength curve is the same as the man or woman
next to you has arms the size of your legs? Do you believe for
a minute your hips are the same width as your next door neighbors, your arms and upper torso are similar in length to every
person in the gym, and your strength is the same as the hulk
wanting to take over the machine you're on? One size fits all
just doesn't deliver much, to anyone!

Realize that weight machines won't fit everybody perfectly.
If it feels wrong, don't use the machine. You may adjust until
you're blue in the face and it'll never be right.

Do weight machines work? Without a doubt. They get similar results as tubing and free weights, when proper load is used.
Results are not dependent on what type of equipment is being
used or whether it's variable resistance. What counts is whether
you're working to fatigue, generally between 6 to 20 reps.

Are multistation gyms really safer than other equipment?
Maybe and maybe not. You always hear they're ideal for begin-

ners because they're so safe, meaning the weight can't fall on you. Yet, I can hear fingers crunching, hair stuck in cable/pulley systems ripping, and joints aching because people have been led to believe machines are perfectly safe. Although weight may never fall on you, be careful around a weight stack.

Machines tend to isolate musculature. They don't require the kind of balance and stabilization needed for every day activity and sport movement. So think about a balanced approach here. If you always train on machines, add some upper body dumbbell exercises, leg squats and lunges to your routine.

And finally, machines generally are not portable, (ever try to fit one in your suitcase?) and they can be a little pricey. Its important to know how to work out with minimal equipment—such as free weights, dumbbells, and tubing—and still optimize your training results. This is especially true if you travel a lot. You never know what will be available to you when you're traveling, and this knowledge keeps you from missing a workout and losing hard won fitness gains!

Elastic Resistance

I know what you're thinking: Come on—tubing? Let's get real and move to the machines and weight! Okay, I know I'm talking about sophisticated rubber bands, but they do the job. You can get them in different thicknesses to let you work harder, some have rotating handles which make them easier to use, they can travel with you, they take up little space, they're inexpensive, and they're effective. And, like free weights, they work with your body because the range of motion is not predetermined and they require some balance as you stretch the tubing. You can hook them to your door (with a door attachment strap), which makes the tubing more versatile.

In other words, you have hundreds of exercises to choose from. If you work against a heavy enough resistance as provided by the tube thickness or by shortening the tube before you perform an exercise, you can get the same results you would from weight machines or dumbbells.

Calisthenics and Lifting Your Own Body Weight

The biggest drawback to using your body weight for strength training exercises is that usually the exercise is too hard or too easy. And, if the amount of effort is just right it doesn't take long before it becomes too easy. Take push-ups or chin-ups as examples. Some people can't do any, others a straining few, and a small number can do them until the cows come home. If the exercise is too hard or too easy, you're probably wasting your time.

Calisthenics and using body weight is not an issue of good or bad. Simply realize their limitations. You can use these types of exercises to maintain some level of strength, and a quick set of push-ups never hurt anyone. To determine their effectiveness, ask this question: can I fatigue the muscles I'm using in 6 to 20 reps? If you can't, you're not optimizing strength results or the use of your time.

Equipment Essentials: The Final Word

Don't believe all the gym stories that attest to a particular piece of equipment's overstated magnificence, effectiveness, and magical qualities. You've got to use the right equipment (defined by your goals), like using it, and use it correctly!

Helpful Hint: How you use the equipment—regardless of cost or lack thereof—is of the utmost importance. Having said that, running a close second, with regard to importance, is the quality of the equipment. Good technique can be short-circuited by equipment that doesn't even have good resale value at a scrap metal yard.

Technically speaking, and from a physiological standpoint, how your body adapts to overload it is not accustomed to (called the training effect) does not change. Neither does the body differentiate between one piece of equipment and the next.

As pointed out earlier, the body only understands effective training and correct overload, regardless of equipment choice.

You need to ask the question, can the equipment I'm using deliver? In other words, principles of overload do not change. If the equipment allows you to exercise harder than your body is used to, and you enjoy doing it on a regular basis, you'll get results. On the other hand, high priced equipment won't do the work for you or necessarily give you better results than less expensive equipment. However, you need to find a balance between useless equipment and high-grade home gym exercise equipment. Obviously, it is you, following the right training guidelines and using correct exercise technique, that optimizes results.

The key is to select equipment that can meet the overload and biomechanical standards of an effective training program, and you don't need to have an unlimited budget to purchase equipment that gets it done. On the other hand, if all the extra features and creature comforts of the top of the line models motivate you to exercise and budget is not a concern, then they're worth the price.

Home Gym Pre-Assessment Questionnaire

What fitness activities have I found to be successful at improving my health and body?

What fitness activities do I find fun and enjoyable and will likely continue for my lifetime?

What, if any, physical limitations do I have (problems such as bad back, knees, shoulders, wrist, or arthritis)?

How would equipment choices complement, or possibly worsen, this condition?

Are my short and long term goals in line with what I am considering purchasing?   yes   no

If yes, how will the equipment purchased help me accomplish my goals?

Will my equipment selections allow me to create balanced workout options that target the major components of fitness, including cardiovascular conditioning, muscular strength and endurance, and flexibility training? If so, how?

Does my home gym equipment offer me the option of cross-training? If so, how?

Will anyone else in my household be using the equipment? If so, will my equipment selection meet their goals and allow them to exercise safely? Will children be using the equipment?

Am I willing to dedicate space in my home for my home gym? If so, have I thought about electrical needs (most home version cardio equipment use standard wall outlets), weight requirements, lighting needs, and floor surfaces?

The room I have available for my home gym is:

_____ ft wide by _____ ft long by _____ ft high.

Checklist for Home Equipment Purchases

This checklist will encourage you to think about information you should consider before buying home fitness equipment. Put a check mark next to each question to which your answer is yes. If you check off the majority of questions in the list, you're on your way to making an informed and useful choice.

❏ **Will I look to a "specialty fitness retailer" or qualified fitness professional to assist me in the research and selection of my home fitness equipment?** (Specialty fitness retailers usually have more qualified sales personnel than mass merchandising sporting good chains. Additionally, many specialty retailers carry commercial grade equipment—such as the equipment clubs use that get heavy use—and high quality home versions of this trustworthy, time tested equipment.)

❏ **Do I understand the high-tech techno talk?** (If not, ask what it means, what it costs you, and how it will help your program. If you get more babble and no helpful answers, it's time to move on.)

❏ **Will I consider each piece of equipment that I purchase with regard to cost, space efficiency, portability, variety, and diversity, and each of these five qualities' importance to my situation?** (Purchasing a bench that declines, lies flat, and inclines is a good example of a piece of equipment that exemplifies these five qualities.)

❏ **Have I tried out every piece of equipment to see if I like it?** (When you shop, wear your workout shoes and comfortable clothes. Spend at least 5 to 10 minutes on every piece of equipment you are considering, and make your own adjustments after the salesperson shows you how. Many specialty retail stores will encourage you to test-ride equipment and have models set up just for this purpose. Or, you can visit local gyms and experience a variety of equipment. Many gyms offer free one week trials you can take advantage of or you can purchase day or short-term memberships so you can try different equipment.)

❏ **Have I talked to other people who have used this equipment?** (Ask the person selling the equipment to give you a list of customers who have bought that particular piece of equipment.)

❏ **Will I really use this equipment or is it going to be a high priced dust collector?**

❏ **Am I committed to buying quality equipment that will last me a lifetime?** (This is in comparison to buying "junk" that will have to be replaced, will frustrate your exercise efforts, and may be unsafe!)

❏ **Is this a piece of equipment that will stand the test of time, or is it trend influenced and destined to fall out of fashion in time?** (Good examples of timeless equipment that never lose their appeal are motorized treadmills and free weights such as dumbbells.)

❏ **Does an equipment purchase come with personal instruction (specialty store retailers usually have knowledgeable sales staff and relationships with personal trainers in your area), a videotaped workout and instruction, other written instructional material?** (Some retailers arrange a free workout with a personal trainer who can show you the ins and outs of your new equipment. Make sure the trainer is certified by a nationally recognized certifying organization.)

❏ **What is the warranty for parts and labor?** (Although the manufacturer's warranty is usually 90 days, ask the retailer if they'll back the equipment for a year. To get a sale, they probably will. Besides, if you're buying a quality piece of equipment, this one-year insurance is probably overkill and the store won't really be at any additional risk. So why not ask for it?)

❏ **Can warranty work, part replacement, repairs, and service be performed locally, or do you have to ship the equipment?** (Specialty retailers generally take care of you since they'd like your repeat business or for you to refer others to them. And, they usually have a full service repair, delivery, and maintenance department.)

❏ **Can I trade the equipment in and upgrade to a higher quality piece?**

❏ **Has the store you're considering purchasing from been in business a number of years?** (Ask the store manager if he could contact any customers who have purchased the equipment you're interested in, and who might be available to talk with you about their purchase.)

❏ **Is the equipment made by a major manufacturer?** (With regard to quality and equipment that will serve you for the long haul, you usually can't go wrong buying brand names.)

❏ **Is the equipment quiet when in use?**

❏ **Is the cushioning made of dense and supportive, yet forgiving, material? Is the external upholstery covering of high quality?** (Compare commercial equipment such as you see in gums with some "cheesy" home exercise equipment and you'll see, and feel the difference. Go for the high-grade equipment. You'll pay more and be glad you did!)

❏ **Do cables and pulleys move smoothly and quietly?**

❏ **What are the safety features?**

❏ **Is the cost of delivery and installation included in the purchase price?** (If not, bargain for it!)

❑ **Is an assembly required after delivery? If it is necessary, is it included in the purchase price?** (If it isn't, ask for it. If a lot of assembly is required, you have the potential for numerous nuts and bolts to work themselves loose over time. Look for pieces that have welded frames and joints and minimal assembly requirements.)

❑ **What is the return policy?** (The manufacturer or retail store should offer, at a minimum, an unconditional 30-day return policy. If for some reason you buy equipment you haven't tried, find out the details of returning the product. Two important questions to ask are whether you have to pay return shipping and whether any of your original purchase price is nonrefundable. Can you trust the company you're buying from? A "free" 30 day trial can cost you some significant money, not to mention the hassle of repacking the junk and sending it back!)

❑ **If a salesperson hurries or tries to push me into a quick decision with answering my questions and encouraging me to try the equipment, will I promptly walk out the door?** (You can do this politely, and the answer should be yes.)

———

The following pages present/reveal the proper way to perform the drills pro players such as Jack Nicklaus, Gary Player, Annika Sorenstam, and Tiger Woods use to play their best golf.

These drills are basic, simple, and proven to produce big improvements in a minimum of time. Follow these instructions and be prepared to save strokes every time you tee up on the golf course.

Leg Press

Focus: Multiple-joint training exercise that works the gluteals, quadriceps, hamstrings, and calves.

Starting Position: Lie on your back on a leg press machine, adjusting the seat/sled to a position where your hips and knees are bent at 90-degree angles. Your feet should be about shoulder-width apart.

Exercise Action: Straighten your knees and hips by pressing down into the platform until they are almost completely straight. Do not lock your knees. Slowly return to the starting position.

Note: A variation of this exercise can be performed with only one leg at a time to focus on each leg independently.

Leg Curl

Focus: Single-joint exercise that primarily works the hamstrings.

Starting Position: Lie on your stomach on the Lying Leg-curl machine. The resistance pad should be adjusted so that it hits you on the lower third of your calf just above the ankle.

Exercise Action: Slowly curl your feet toward your buttocks. Slowly return the weights to the starting position. Your knees should not hyperextend in the starting position.

Squat

Focus: Multiple-joint exercise that works many muscles, including the gluteals, quadriceps, hamstrings, back extensors, and calves.

Starting Position: Stand with your feet parallel to your shoulders; hold dumbbells in your hands resting at your sides, or hold a medicine ball placed behind your neck and stabilized with both hands.

Exercise Action: Bend your legs in a slow, controlled manner until your knees are at a 90-degree angle with your thighs parallel to the ground. As you bend, keep your head up and look straight ahead, and keep your chest out, and back flat. Your weight should be back toward the middle and rear of your feet, not on your toes. Return to the starting position, keeping your head up and back flat.

Note: If you have knee problems or a history of knee problems, bend your knees only 45 to 60 degrees, as you can tolerate.

Front Lunge

Focus: Multiple-joint exercise that works most muscles in the lower extremities and trunk.

Starting Position: Stand with your feet six to eight inches apart; hold a dumbbell or place a medicine ball comfortably behind your neck and stabilize it with both hands.

Exercise Action: Take a large step forward and position your body over your front leg. Bend your front knee so it is in line with or slightly in front of the ankle joint and does not project beyond the front of your shoe. Return to the starting position by pushing your weight backward and straightening your front leg. You may need to take a few small steps to return your leg to the starting position. Keep your trunk erect during the exercise by looking straight ahead and keeping your chest out. Alternate legs.

Variation 1: Crossover lunge: Instead of stepping straight forward, step out with your front leg in a 45-degree diagonal (move the left leg in a crossing direction in front of your right leg and foot). Alternate between the right and left legs, using crossover diagonal pattern.

Variation 2: Side Lunge: Step directly to your right or left side, sinking into a squat position as shown. Alternate between the left and right sides. If you have knee problems, bend the knee only 30 to 45 degrees to decrease stress.

Calf Raise

Focus: Develops the gastrocnemius and soleus (calf muscles).

Starting Position: Stand with your feet six to eight inches apart; hold dumbbells in each hand or place a medicine ball comfortably behind your head and stabilize with both hands.

Exercise Action: Keeping your knees straight and trunk upright, raise your heels off the ground until you are standing on the balls of your feet. Slowly return to the starting position. Begin this exercise standing on the floor but progress to performing it with your toes on a step or on the platform of an exercise machine. This position allows the heels to drop below the balls of the feet when you start and allows you to exercise through a larger range of motion.

Crunch

Focus: Develops power for all strokes. A strong trunk (rectus abdominis) is the source of many movements and allows the upper body to stay synchronized with the lower body.

Starting Position: Lie on your back with knees bent and feet flat on the floor. Hold your hands behind your head, with the elbows to the sides or crossed resting on top of your chest. Refrain from pulling your head forward with your hands.

Exercise Action: Curl the upper body from the floor, including the head and the shoulders, until you can feel the abdominal muscles contracting. The upper body should be off the ground by about three inches at the shoulder blades. Lower until the shoulder blades touch the ground and repeat.

Crossover Crunch

Focus: Strengthens the internal and external oblique muscles of the trunk, which are responsible for trunk rotation.

Starting Position: Lie on your back with one knee bent and the foot flat on the floor. The opposite knee is bent so the heel rests on the other knee. Hold your hands behind your head with elbows out to the sides. Refrain from pulling your head forward with your hands.

Exercise Action: Curl the upper body so the elbow opposite the elevated knee moves toward it diagonally. Repeat this movement on the opposite side.

Trunk Circles

Focus: Develops the entire abdomen and trunk. This exercise requires more strength than the basic abdominal exercises.

Starting Position: Lie on your back with your hips and knees bent at 90 degrees. Hold your arms and hands behind your head with elbows out to the sides. Refrain from pulling the head forward with the hands.

Exercise Action: Touch the left elbow to the right knee and vice versa. Alternate touches without allowing the knees to rest.

Reverse Sit-up

Focus: Works the rectus abdominis through a full range of motion with little use of the iliopsoas (hip flexors).

Starting Position: Lie on your back, raise your feet and place them on a box or bench. Hold your hands behind your head with elbows out to the side. Refrain from pulling your head forward with your hands.

Exercise Action: Curl up your body and attempt to touch your chest to the thighs.

Hip Raises

Focus: Develops rectus abdominis strength.

Starting Position: Lie on your back with your hips elevated and legs straight in the air. Place arms and hands out to the sides for stability or under the lower back for support.

Exercise Action: Raise your hips off the ground and point the toes toward the ceiling while flexing the abdominal wall. Slowly lower your hips to the ground and repeat.

Diagonal Sit-up

Focus: Targets the oblique muscles of the trunk.

Starting Position: Secure your feet on the floor—with a partner or under a bench—with your knees bent and your body flat against the floor. Place both arms on the same side.

Exercise Action: Bring the arms up and across the body using the trunk to raise and twist to the opposite side. Perform a diagonal movement, alternating sides.

Russian Twist

Focus: Works the obliques of the trunk.

Starting Position: Secure your feet on the floor, with your knees bent and body leaning back at a 45-degree angle. Hold your arms straight out from the shoulders so they are parallel with the thighs. Hold a club or weights to increase the resistance of the exercise.

Exercise Action: Rotate side to side, turning the shoulders until the arms are at a 90-degree angle with the body. Make a full twist to the opposite side. Over and back is one repetition.

Hip Rotation

Focus: Develops strength in the rectus abdominis, obliques, and iliopsoas.

Starting Position: Lie on your back with your hips flexed and knees extended. Place arms and hands out to the sides for stability.

Exercise Action: Rotate hips and trunk to one side until they touch the ground. Keeping knees together, rotate them all the way over until they touch on the other side. You have done one full rotation when you have touched both sides.

Back Extension

Focus: Helps prevent overuse injuries or chronic lower back pain by targeting the erector spinae muscles along the spinal column.

Starting Position: Lie flat on the floor with the arms fully extended above the head.

Exercise Action: Lift both arms and both legs simultaneously. Hold this position for one to five seconds and return to the start position. A variation might include lifting the right arm and left leg, followed by lifting the left arm and right leg.

Pec Dec/Pec Flye

Focus: To strengthen the center pectoral muscles without involving your triceps. These muscles are used during the backswing.

Starting Position: Have a seat on the pec dec/pec flye machine with your arms about parallel to the floor and your back flat against the back rest.

Exercise Action: Pull the pads together as far as possible, pause, and then slowly return to the start. It's important not to let your elbows extend beyond a point where they are in line with your shoulders. Such an extreme range of motion may cause injury to your shoulder.

Pull Over Toss

Focus: To develop upper body strength and power.

Starting Position: Lie faceup on the floor with your arms extended behind you.

Exercise Action: Hold a medicine ball with your hands facing each other. Have a partner stand about 10 feet in front of you to serve as a catcher.

Pull the ball overhead and to your chest while moving into a sitting position. Perform a chest pass to your partner. Remain in the upright position to catch the toss-back from your partner. Repeat for the required number of repetions. To make the exercise harder have your partner stand farther back.

Hip Roll

Focus: To strengthen your trunk by developing your lower abdominal muscles.

Starting Position: Lie face up on the floor with your hands at your sides or under your tail bone.

Exercise Action: Press your lower back to the floor and try to maintain this position with your back throughout the exercise (start). Keeping your knees bent, lift your legs toward your chest, then slowly lower to the start.

To increase the difficulty of this exercise, perform it at a slower pace, place your hands behind your head, or lie faceup on an incline sit-up board.

Knee Pull-in

Focus: To strengthen your trunk by developing your abdominal muscles.

Starting Position: Lie faceup across a sturdy bench with your bottom at the edge of the bench.

Exercise Action: Pull your knees to your chest and your chest toward your knee (finish). Reverse the procedure to return to the start. Do not allow your head to drop below horizontal any time during the exercise.

Rotator-Cuff Program

The following exercises work your rotator-cuff muscles. These exercises are performed with rubber tubing. You should initially perform them with tubing using one or two pounds of resistance. If you use a heavier resistance you may compensate and perform the exercise using larger muscle groups that are already developed. Even the strongest, largest golfers use a maximum of four or five pounds for these exercises.

You can purchase your rubber tubing or Thera-band from physical therapy clinics and fitness dealers. You can use the medium (blue colored) or medium heavy (black colored) tubes for your rotator cuff strengthening.

External Shoulder Rotation

Focus: Works the external shoulder rotators, scapular stabilizers, and posterior deltoid.

Starting Position: Lie on your stomach on a table with arm hanging down toward the floor, holding dumbbells in your hands.

Exercise Action: With the thumb pointed outward, raise the arm back toward the hip. Slowly lower the arm and repeat.

External Shoulder Rotation with Tubing

Focus: Develops external rotation strength.

Starting Position: Secure rubber tubing to a doorknob at about waist height. Stand sideways to the door with the lead arm away from the door. Place a small, rolled towel under the lead arm.

Exercise Action: Hold the rubber tubing in your hand and start with the hand close to the abdomen. Rotate the hand and forearm away from the abdomen until the hand and forearm are straight out in front, pulling on the tube for resistance. Return to the starting position and repeat. Keep your elbow at a 90-degree angle throughout the exercise. You can place your opposite hand under your elbow to support the arm if needed.

External Shoulder Rotation with Abduction

Focus: Works the rotator cuff in golf-swing-specific position.

Starting Position: Secure the rubber tubing to a doorknob at about waist height. Stand facing the door with your shoulder bent 90 degrees, about 30 degrees in front of you on a diagonal. Use your opposite hand to support your upper arm.

Exercise Action: Hold the tubing in your hand and rotate your hand back until it reaches nearly vertical. Return to the starting position and repeat.

Internal Shoulder Rotation

Focus: Develops internal rotation strength.

Starting Position: Secure the rubber tubing to a doorknob at about waist height. Stand sideways to the door with the lead arm close to the door. Place a small, rolled towel under the lead arm.

Exercise Action: Hold the rubber tubing in the lead hand and start with the hand and forearm straight out in front of you. Rotate the hand in toward the abdomen. Return to the starting position and repeat. Keep your elbow at a 90-degree angle throughout the exercise. You can place your opposite hand under your elbow to support the arm if needed.

Additional Upper Body Exercises

Seated Row

Focus: Develops the rhomboids, trapezius, posterior deltoid, and biceps.

Starting Position: Sit with your knees slightly bent and your hands holding a cord or band device, cable machine, or seated row machine.

Exercise Action: While keeping the upper chest erect and not leaning backward, pull band handles toward the chest and upper abdomen area. Keep the elbows close to your sides. Slowly return to the start position and repeat.

Lat Pulldown

Focus: Develops the latissimus dorsi and biceps muscles.

Starting Position: Using a Lat Pulldown machine, overhead cable, or rubber tubing, reach upward to grasp the handles with a wide grip.

Exercise Action: Pull down the bar, cable, or tubing, bringing the bar in front of you toward the middle of your chest. Slowly return the bar to the starting position with control and repeat.

Chest Press

Focus: Develops the pectoralis major/minor, serratus anterior, triceps, and anterior deltoid.

Starting Position: Lie on your back on a narrow bench with the arms externally rotated at a 90-degree angle to the torso. The exercise may be performed with dumbbells or barbells.

Exercise Action: While keeping the wrist directly over the elbows and not locking the elbows, extend your hands toward the ceiling. As you extend your hands upward, round your shoulders pushing your hands as far away from you as you can. This extra motion works the serratus anterior muscle, which supports your shoulder blade while you play golf.

Biceps Curl

Focus: Works the biceps brachii, brachialis, and brachioradialis.

Starting Position: Stand holding a dumbbell in your hand with your feet shoulder-width apart.

Exercise Action: Keeping your shoulder at your side, bend your elbow and bring the weight toward your shoulder. If you have chosen the weight correctly, you should not be arching your back or leaning backward during the exercise. Slowly return the weight to the starting position, making sure you don't hyperextend or lock your elbow.

Prone Flys

Focus: Develops the posterior deltoid, rhomboids, and trapezius.

Starting Position: Lie on your stomach on a narrow bench with your feet off the ground.

Exercise Action: With dumbbells in hand, extend your arms from your sides at a 90-degree angle. They should be pointed toward the ground. While maintaining a right angle at the shoulder raise your arms until they are nearly parallel to the ground.

Wrist Curls: Extensors

Focus: Develops the wrist and finger extensors.

Starting Position: Holding a pair of dumbbells, sit in a chair with the elbow bent and forearm resting on a table or over your knee. Let the wrist and hand hang over the edge. Turn the hand so the palm is down.

Exercise Action: Stabilize the forearm with the opposite hand, and slowly curl your wrist and hand upward. Be sure to move only at your wrist, not at your elbow. Raise your hand slowly, hold for a count, and slowly lower it. Repeat. Switch arms.

Wrist Curls: Flexors

Focus: Develops the wrist and forearm flexors.

Starting Position: Holding a pair of dumbbells, sit in a chair with elbows bent and forearm resting on a table or over your knee. Let the wrist and hand hang over the edge. Turn the hand so the palm is up.

Exercise Action: Stabilize the forearm with the opposite hand, and slowly curl your wrist and hand upward. Be sure to move only at your wrist, not at your elbow. Raise your hand slowly, hold for a count, and slowly lower it. Repeat. Switch arms.

Forearm Pronation

Focus: Develops the forearm pronators.

Starting Position: Sit in a chair with the elbow bent and forearm resting on a table or your knee. Let the wrist and hand hang over the edge. Using a dumbbell with a weight at only one end (i.e., hammer), begin the exercise with the palm upward so the handle is horizontal.

Exercise Action: Slowly rotate your forearm and wrist so the weight is in the upright (vertical) position. Hold for a count, then slowly return to the starting position. Switch arms.

Forearm Supination

Focus: Develops the forearm supinators.

Starting Position: Sit in a chair with your elbow bent and forearm resting on a table or your knee. Let the wrist and hand hang over the edge. Using a dumbbell with weight at only one end (i.e., hammer), begin the exercise with the palm down.

Exercise Action: Slowly rotate your forearm and wrist until the weight is in the upright position. Hold for a count, then slowly return to the starting position. Switch arms.

Radial Deviation

Focus: Develops the muscles that stabilize the wrist during golf.

Starting Position: Stand with your arm at your side and grasp a dumbbell with the weight on only one end (i.e., hammer). The weighted end should be in front in a neutral position (thumb pointing straight ahead of you).

Exercise Action: Slowly raise and lower the weight through a comfortable range of motion. All the movement should occur at the wrist with no elbow or shoulder joint movement. You will not be able to exercise through a large arc of movement. Repeat. Switch arms.

Ulnar Deviation

Focus: Develops the muscles that stabilize the wrist during golf.

Starting Position: Stand with your arm at your side, and grasp a dumbbell with weight on only one end (i.e., hammer). The weighted end should be behind your exercising hand.

Exercise Action: With your forearm in the neutral position (thumb pointing straight ahead of you), slowly raise and lower the weight through a comfortable range of motion. All the movement should occur at your wrist with no elbow or shoulder joint movement. You will not be able to exercise through a large arc of movement. Repeat. Switch arms.

Plyometric Medicine Ball Program

These exercises develop power in the upper body. They use a medicine ball for resistance and require explosive movement patterns. Typically, you can do them with a four- to six-pound medicine ball. You can increase the weight of the ball when the workout becomes too easy. Begin with sets of 20 to 25 repetitions of each exercise, and advance to performing sets until you get fatigued. If you can perform more than 50 repetitions without fatigue, you should increase the weight of the ball.

Chest Pass

Focus: Works the pectorals, triceps, and scapular stabilizers.

Starting Position: Stand eight to ten feet from a partner. Hold the ball in front of the chest.

Exercise Action: Pass the ball to the partner. When you receive the ball from your partner, try to catch and release it back to your partner as quickly as possible.

Overhead Toss

Focus: Develops the latissimus dorsi and triceps muscles.

Starting Position: Stand eight to ten feet from a partner. Hold the medicine ball directly overhead.

Exercise Action: Toss the ball to your partner. When you receive the ball from your partner, try to catch and release it back to your partner as quickly as possible.

Downswing Toss

Focus: Develops the muscles used in the downswing.

Starting Position: Stand eight to ten feet from a partner. Hold the ball with both hands at your downswing side.

Exercise Action: Turn just as you would during the golf swing. Pass the ball to your partner, mimicking an aggressive downswing. When you receive the ball back from your partner, try to catch and release it back to your partner as quickly as possible.

Backswing Toss

Focus: Develops muscles used in the backswing.

Starting Position: Stand eight to ten feet from a partner. Hold the ball with both hands at your backswing side.

Exercise Action: Step and turn, just as you would to make your backswing, taking the ball back like a club. Pass the ball to your partner, mimicking a powerful backswing. When you receive the ball from your partner, try to catch and release it back to your partner as quickly as possible.

Woodchops or Side Throws

Focus: Emphasizes the trunk rotation and development of the obliques and rectus abdominis.

Starting Position: Stand eight to ten feet from a partner, sideways. Hold the ball at shoulder height with both hands.

Exercise Action: Throw the ball using a sideways and slightly downward movement pattern to your partner. When you receive the ball from your partner, try to catch and release it back to your partner as quickly as possible.

Standing Trunk Twist

Focus: Develops the trunk and lower back musculature: rectus, erector spinae, obliques, and gluteals.

Starting Position: Stand back to back with a partner, with one or two feet between you and your partner. Hold the ball at waist height.

Exercise Action: Hand the ball to your partner by rotating to the right and your partner rotating to the left. The partner will then take the ball and rotate to the opposite side as you receive the ball by rotating to your left. Continue this pattern for a desired number of repetitions; then repeat this exercise by changing directions.

Sit-ups with Partner Toss

Focus: Develops the rectus abdominis using a more explosive power-oriented format.

Starting Position: Lie on your back with your knees bent 90 degrees and feet on the floor. Hold a medicine ball in both hands over your chest. Have a partner stand three to five feet from your feet.

Exercise Action: Sit up and pass the ball to your partner as you come up. Continue the upward motion of your sit-up, and instruct your partner to pass the ball to you as you return to the starting position. Try to absorb the weight of the ball without gaining speed.

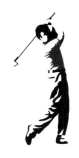

CHAPTER FIVE

Heart of a Champion:
Aerobic and Endurance Exercises

How important is endurance in golf? Imagine walking 18 holes, anywhere from four to five miles on average, and being out of breath before and after every shot. Without overall endurance you cannot play optimal golf. Now add carrying a bag to the equation. The physical effort you use, unless you are in good shape, drains your mental and physical energy away from your game.

Golf is not a game of endurance like running a marathon or cycling. But fitness is important in golf. It may not improve your swing, but it will reduce your overall fatigue and improve your mental game.

Does Playing Golf Build Endurance?

The short answer is no. Walking a round of 18 holes at a normal pace is not challenging enough to increase your aerobic capacity, because you are walking, stopping, and hitting the ball, then waiting and walking again. You are not exercising hard enough or long enough to improve your endurance beyond a minor level.

Exactly how much endurance is required or developed depends on a number of factors: how fit you are, how much your bag weighs, the terrain of the course, and the temperature and humidity at the time you are walking.

Aerobic Endurance and Golf Performance

You will play better if you have a finely tuned, well-conditioned, fuel-efficient body. A higher-than-average aerobic fitness level increases your overall energy level. Being better conditioned will allow you to keep your focus on the course because you will not be physically tired and you will be able to put your energy into shot selection and course management.

You should train at a level that is 5- to 10-percent higher than what it takes for you to complete a round of golf. Your extra energy can be used in other parts of your game, you will feel stronger, swing better, and be a more confident and focused player. Once you are in proper condition, you will never have to worry about a round of golf tiring you to the point where it affects your game. Since your swing relies on muscular endurance, which improves with your aerobic capacity, your swing will be more consistent.

Golf is as tough mentally as physically. Every shot you take requires focus that must be repeated over the course of four or more hours of golf. Concentration requires real physical energy. The more fit golfer can maintain energy levels and focus so that the putt made on the final hole is as smooth and balanced as the one made on the practice green several hours earlier.

Aerobic Training for Golf

For an exercise activity to stress the aerobic system, golfers need to adhere to several basic concepts: Aerobic exercise training activities typically involve large muscle groups, are repetitive, and include continuous repeated or cycled exertion. Examples of this are running, swimming, stair climbing, and biking.

Additional characteristics of aerobic exercise include frequency, duration, and intensity. One key document used when recommending aerobic exercise is produced by the American College of Sports Medicine (ACSM).

Exercise Variables

How do you set up a training program to gain aerobic fitness for golf? Your golf-conditioning program consists of four variables:

- **Intensity:** the amount of effort used during the exercise. It is measured in the amount of calories burned per hour or per minute. It can also be measured by the heart rate during exercise, your perceived exertion, and calories burned per hour. You should work at 60 to 85 percent of your maximum heart rate.

- **Duration:** the length of time spent per training session. In general, it is recommended that 20 minutes at the proper intensity is needed to increase aerobic endurance.

- **Frequency:** the number of sessions per week. Building aerobic fitness takes a minimum of three sessions per week if you are new to exercise. To significantly improve your endurance you may need four or more sessions per week. Keeping a certain fitness level once it has been reached requires three training sessions per week. However, if you walk the course more than three times per week you can cut down to two weekly aerobic sessions once you have reached your target conditioning goal.

- **Mode:** the type of exercise you choose. Good choices for the golfer are walking, running/jogging, cycling, stair stepping, slide-board training, and swimming. If your goal is to enhance your golf performance, then a mix of modes will produce the best gains in the shortest amount of time.

How Hard Should You Train?

Improvements in cardiovascular fitness occur in the training zone of 60 to 85 percent of your maximum heart rate (MHR). No matter what exercise you choose, the intensity must be at this level.

Your MHR is roughly 220 minus your age. For example, a 40-year-old man would have an MHR of 180 beats per minute (bpm). So his training zone is 180 × .60, to get 108 beats per minute.

What should your heart rate be? People new to exercises should work at the low end of the training zone of 55 percent to 70 percent of MHR; golfers of average fitness and some exercise experience work at 70 percent to 85 percent; and trained athletes can train as high as 90 percent of MHR.

Always check with your physician before starting an exercise program, especially if you are over forty, have significant risk factors for heart disease, or have symptoms of heart disease.

Adding Aerobic Fitness to a Golfer's Program

Improving and maintaining aerobic fitness levels is an important part in the overall training program for golfers. It is recommended that players with low levels of aerobic fitness be identified using the fitness testing guidelines in chapter two. Depending on the degree of need in the individual's training program, aerobic exercise is an important activity to include. Several factors are important to consider before adding aerobic training to your program:

- **Timing:** Do not fatigue yourself with aerobic exercise before a skill practice session. Do aerobic training after skill-oriented, golf-specific training and on days of light training of other components.

- **Frequency:** As with other types of exercise training, start aerobic training gradually; for example, complete aerobic activities one or two times per week along with other aspects of training and progress based on your needs.

- **Variety:** Choose an aerobic training activity that you will enjoy. Use cross training with aerobic training to avoid boredom, encourage development of multiple muscle groups, and increase enjoyment.

- **Testing:** Use testing to measure aerobic-fitness levels and gauge improvement (see chapter two). Excessive aerobic training may invite overuse injuries and take valuable training time from skill-oriented golf training.

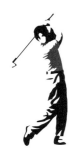

CHAPTER SIX

Stroke-Saver Workout:
Sample Training Programs

I have taken the liberty to share with you a program similar to what my tour players follow. Golf has become such a big-money sport at every level, players like to keep secret what helps them perform better. But what won't remain secret for long is how much longer and accurate your drives are, how much better your putting is, and how much lower your scores are on a regular basis.

The program is divided into three four-week blocks. Each block progresses to the next block.

Block 1: Strength-Endurance Workouts

You should perform Block 1 workouts at least two but prefer-ably three days a week for the first four weeks of the Golfer's Stroke-Saver Workout program. If you train three days per week, the workouts for Days 1 and 3 are the same.

Note: A complex is a type of set in which two exercises are performed alternately (instead of the conventional method of per-forming all of the sets of one exercise before moving to the next exercise). A circuit is a set in which several exercises are performed in sequence.

After every workout, you need to perform five to ten min-utes of the post-workout stretches from chapter three.

Also, you will supplement your Block 1 workouts with aer-obic training preferably performed on the days you are resting from the workouts.

Block 1: Preparation Phase Workouts

Duration: four weeks
Workouts: three per week using training components from
   chapter four

Supplementary Work
Arobic training from chapter five

Preparation Phase

Block 1: Day 1

Note: Unless otherwise stated, rest one minute after every set;
   r=reps; s=sets; sec=seconds.

1. **Standard warm-up**

2. **Plyometrics and medicine ball**

   Overhead Toss: 15r × 2s

   Weight: _____

   Woodchops or Side Throws: 15r × 2s

   Weight: _____

3. **Weight training, circuit 1 (2s)** Week 1 40% Max; Week 2
   50% Max; Week 3 60% Max; Week 4 70% Max

   Squat: 10–15r; down in four sec, no
                             pause, up at moderate speed

   Weight: _____

   Front Lunge: 10–15r; down in four sec, no
                             pause, up at moderate speed

   Weight: _____

   Side Lunge: 10–15r; down in four sec, no
                             pause, up at moderate speed

   Weight: _____

Calf Raise (machine):	10–15r; up at moderate speed, no pause, down in four sec
Weight: _____	

Rest two to three minutes after each set

4. Weight training, circuit 2 (2s) Week 1 40% Max; Week 2 50% Max; Week 3 60% Max; Week 4 70% Max

Prone fly:	10–15r; up at moderate speed, no pause, down in 4 sec
Weight: _____	
Seated row:	0–15r; up at moderate speed, no pause, down in 4 sec
Weight: _____	
Lat pulldown:	10–15r; up at moderate speed, no pause, down in 4 sec
Weight: _____	
Biceps Curl:	10–15r; up at moderate speed, no pause, down in 4 sec
Weight: _____	

Rest two to three minutes after each set

5. Abdominal circuit (1s) (using weights)

Crossover Crunch:	25r
Russian Twist:	10r (each side); down in four sec, no pause, up at moderate pace
Weight: _____	
Reverse Sit-up:	25r
Hip Raises:	15r
Back Extension:	10r x 2s; up at moderate speed, no pause, down in four sec
Weight: _____	

6. **Wrist-forearm circuit (1s) (using weights)** Week 1 40% Max; Week 2 50% Max; Week 3 60% Max; Week 4 70% Max

Wrist Curls: Flexors: 20r; moderate speed

   Weight: _____

Wrist Curls: Extensors: 20r; moderate speed

   Weight: _____

Forearm Pronation: 20r; moderate speed

   Weight: _____

Forearm Supination: 20r; moderate speed

   Weight: _____

Ulnar Deviation: 20r; moderate speed

   Weight: _____

Radial Deviation: 20r; moderate speed

   Weight: _____

7. **Rotator-cuff circuit (2s) (using weights or tubing)**

External Shoulder Rotation: 20r; moderate speed

   Weight: _____

Internal Shoulder Rotation   20r; moderate speed

   Weight: _____

External Shoulder Rotation   20r; moderate speed
with Abduction:

   Weight: _____

Additional work: Post-workout stretches

Supplementary aerobics: Week 1–4 (see chapter five)
Aerobic Training
Frequency: three sessions per week at intensity or 65 to 75% MHR for 20 minutes
Mode: Vary mode each time you work out. Choose from treadmill walking/running, stationary bike, stair climbing, or aerobic riding.

Preparation Phase

Block 1: Day 2

Note: Unless otherwise stated, rest 1 minute after every set, r=reps; s=sets; sec=seconds.

1. **Standard warm-up**

2. **Plyometrics and medicine ball**

    Overhead Toss: 15r x 2s

        Weight: _____

    Woodchops or Side Throws: 15r x 2s

        Weight: _____

3. **Weight training circuit, 1 (2s)** Week 1 40% Max; Week 2 50% Max; Week 3 60% Max; Week 4 70% Max

    Front Lunge: 10–15r; down in four sec, no pause, up at moderate speed

        Weight: _____

    Hip Raises: 10–15r; down in four sec, no pause, up at moderate speed

        Weight: _____

    Leg Curl: 10–15r; down in four sec, no pause, up at moderate speed

        Weight: _____

    Calf Raise: 20r; up at moderate speed, no pause, down in four sec

        Weight: _____

Rest two to three minutes after each set

4. Weight training, circuit 2 (2s) Week 1 40% Max; Week 2 50% Max; Week 3 60% Max; Week 4 70% Max

Chest Press:	10–15r; up at moderate speed, no pause, down in four sec
Weight: _____	
Lat Pulldown:	10–15r; up at moderate speed, no pause, down in four sec
Weight: _____	
Pec dec:	10–15r; up at moderate speed, no pause, down in four sec
Weight: _____	
Seated row:	10–15r; up at moderate speed, no pause, down in four sec
Weight: _____	

Rest two to three minutes after each set

5. Abdominal circuit (1s) (using weights)

Crossover Crunch:	25r
Russian Twist:	10r (each side); down in four sec, no pause, up at moderate speed
Weight: _____	
Reverse Sit-up:	25r
Hip Raises:	15r
Back Extension:	10r x 2s; up at moderate speed, no pause, down in four sec
Weight: _____	

6. Wrist-forearm circuit (1s) (using weights) Week 1 40% Max; Week 2 50% Max; Week 3 60% Max; Week 4 70% Max

Wrist Curls: Flexors:	20r; moderate speed
Weight: _____	

Wrist Curls: Extensors: 20r; moderate speed
>   *Weight:* _____

Forearm Pronation: 20r; moderate speed
>   *Weight:* _____

Forearm Supination: 20r; moderate speed
>   *Weight:* _____

Ulnar Deviation: 20r; moderate speed
>   *Weight:* _____

Radial Deviation: 20r; moderate speed
>   *Weight:* _____

7. **Rotator-cuff circuit (2s)** Maximum weight of 5 lbs.

External Shoulder Rotation: 20r; moderate speed
>   *Weight:* _____

Internal Shoulder Rotation: 20r; moderate speed
>   *Weight:* _____

External Shoulder Rotation
with Abduction: 20r; moderate speed
>   *Weight:* _____

Additional work: Post-workout stretches

Supplementary aerobics: Week 1–4 (see chapter five)
Aerobic Training
Frequency: three sessions per week at intensity or 65 to 75%
MHR for 20 minutes
Mode: Vary mode each time you work out. Choose from
treadmill walking/running, stationary bike, stair climbing,
or aerobic riding.

Preparation Phase

Block 1: Day 3

Note: Unless otherwise stated, rest 1 minute after every set,
r=reps; s=sets; sec=seconds.

1. **Standard warm-up**

2. **Plyometrics and medicine ball**

   Overhead Toss: 15r x 2s

   > *Weight:* _____

   Woodchops or Side Throws: 15r x 2s

   > *Weight:* _____

3. **Weight training, circuit 1 (2s)** Week 1 40% Max; Week 2
   50% Max; Week 3 60% Max; Week 4 70% Max

   Squat: 10–15r; down in four sec, no
                                 pause, up at moderate speed

   > *Weight:* _____

   Front Lunge: 10–15r; down in four sec, no
                                 pause, up at moderate speed

   > *Weight:* _____

   Side Lunge: 10–15r; down in four sec, no
                                 pause, up at moderate speed

   > *Weight:* _____

   Calf Raise: 10–15r; up at moderate speed,
                                 no pause, down in four sec

   > *Weight:* _____

Rest two to three minutes after each set

4. **Weight training, circuit 2 (2s)** Week 1 40% Max; Week 2
   50% Max; Week 3 60% Max; Week 4 70% Max

Prone Fly:	10–15r; up at moderate speed, no pause, down in four sec
Weight: _____	
Seated Row:	10–15r; up at moderate speed, no pause, down in four sec
Weight: _____	
Lat Pulldown:	10–15r; up at moderate speed, no pause, down in four sec
Weight: _____	
Biceps Curl:	10–15r; up at moderate speed, no pause, down in four sec
Weight: _____	

   Rest two to three minutes after each set

5. **Abdominal circuit (1s) (using weights)**

Crossover crunch:	25r
Russian Twist:	10r (each side); down in four sec, no pause, up at moderate speed
Weight: _____	
Reverse Sit-up:	25r
Hip Raises:	15r
Back Extension:	10r x 2s; up at moderate speed, no pause, down in four sec
Weight: _____	

6. **Wrist-forearm circuit (1s) (using weights)** Week 1 40% Max;
   Week 2 50% Max; Week 3 60% Max; Week 4 70% Max

Wrist Curls: Flexors:	20r; moderate speed
Weight: _____	

Wrist Curls: Extensors: 20r; moderate speed

> *Weight:* _____

Forearm Pronation: 20r; moderate speed

> *Weight:* _____

Forearm Supination: 20r; moderate speed

> *Weight:* _____

Ulnar Deviation: 20r; moderate speed

> *Weight:* _____

Radial Deviation: 20r; moderate speed

> *Weight:* _____

Additional work: Post-workout stretches

Supplementary aerobics: Week 1–4 (see chapter five)
Aerobic Training
Frequency: three sessions per week at intensity or 65 to 75%
MHR for 20 minutes
Mode: Vary mode each time you work out. Choose from
treadmill walking/running, stationary bike, stair climbing,
or aerobic riding.

Block 2: Precompetitive Phase Workouts

You should perform Block 2 workouts at least two but preferably three days a week for the first four weeks of the Golfer's
Stroke-Saver Workout program. If you train three days per
week, the workouts for Days 1 and 3 are the same.

Note: A complex is a type of set in which two exercises are
performed alternately (instead of in the conventional method
of performing all sets of one exercise before moving to the next
exercise). A circuit is a set in which several exercises are
performed in sequence.

After every workout you need to perform five to ten minutes of the post-workout stretches from chapter three.

Also, you will supplement your Block 2 workouts with aerobic training preferably performed on the days you are resting from the workouts.

Block 2: Precompetitive Phase Workouts

Duration: four weeks
Workouts: three per week using training components from chapter four

Supplementary Work
Aerobic training from chapter five

Precompetitive Phase

Block 2: Day 1

Note: Unless otherwise stated, rest one minute after every set; r=reps; s=sets; sec=seconds.

1. **Standard warm-up**

2. **Weight training (conventional method) (2s)** Week 1 60% Max; Week 2 65% Max; Week 3 70% Max; Week 4 75% Max

Leg Press:	10r; up at max speed, pause for one second, down in three sec
Weight: _____	
Back Extension:	10r; up at max speed, pause for one second, down in three sec
Weight: _____	
Lat Pulldown:	10r; up at max speed, pause for one second, down in three sec
Weight: _____	

| Front Raises: | 10r; up at max speed, pause for one second, down in three sec |

Weight: _____

| External Shoulder Rotations: | 10–15r; moderate speed |

Weight: _____

Rest two to three minutes after each set

3. Plyometrics and medicine ball

| Chest Pass: | 15r x 3s |

Weight: _____

| Woodchops or Side Throws | 15r x 2s |

Weight: _____

4. Abdominal circuit (2s) (using weights)

Crossover Crunch:	25r (each side)
Seated Trunk Circles:	15r
Reverse Sit-up:	25r
Diagonal Sit-up:	12r
Russian Twist:	10r (each side); down in three sec, pause one sec, up at max speed

Weight: _____

5. Wrist-forearm circuit (1s) (using weights) Week 1 40% Max; Week 2 50% Max; Week 3 60% Max; Week 4 70% Max

| Wrist Curls: Flexors: | 20r; moderate speed |

Weight: _____

| Wrist Curls: Extension: | 20r; moderate speed |

Weight: _____

Forearm Pronation: 20r; moderate speed
    Weight: _____

Forearm Supination: 20r; moderate speed
    Weight: _____

Ulnar Deviation: 20r; moderate speed
    Weight: _____

Radial Deviation: 20r; moderate speed
    Weight: _____

6. **Rotator-cuff circuit (2s)** Maximum weight of 5 lbs.

External Shoulder Rotation: 20r; moderate speed
    Weight: _____

Internal Shoulder Rotation: 20r; moderate speed
    Weight: _____

External Shoulder Rotation
with Abduction: 20r; moderate speed
    Weight: _____

Additional work: Post-workout stretches

Supplementary aerobics: Week 4–8 (see chapter five)
Aerobic Training
Frequency: three sessions per week at intensity or 65 to 75%
   MHR for 20 minutes
Mode: Vary mode each time you work out. Choose from
   treadmill walking/running, stationary bike, stair climbing,
   or aerobic riding.

Precompetitive Phase

Block 2: Day 2

Note: Unless otherwise stated, rest one minute after every set; r=reps; s=sets; sec=seconds.

1. **Standard warm-up**

2. **Weight training, circuit 1 (2s)** Week 1 60% Max; Week 2 65% Max; Week 3 70% Max; Week 4 75% Max

   | Front Lunge: | 10r (each leg); down in three sec, pause one sec, up at max speed |

   Weight: _____

   | Crossover Lunge: | 10r (each leg); down in three sec, pause one sec, up at max speed |

   Weight: _____

   | Side Lunge: | 10r (each leg); down in three sec, pause one sec, up at max speed |

   Weight: _____

   Rest two to three minutes after each set

3. **Weight training, circuit 2 (2s)** Week 1 60% Max; Week 2 65% Max; Week 3 70% Max; Week 4 75% Max

   | Chest press: | 10r; down in three sec, pause one sec, up at max speed |

   Weight: _____

   | Prone Fly: | 10r; down in three sec, pause one sec, up at max speed |

   Weight: _____

Lat Pulldown: 10r; down in three sec, pause one sec, up at max speed

Weight: _____

Front raise (dumbbells):   10r; up in three sec, pause one sec, down at max speed

Weight: _____

Rest two to three minutes after each set

4. Plyometrics and medicine ball

Chest Pass: 15r x 3s

Weight: _____

Woodchops or Side Throws: 15r x 2s

Weight: _____

5. Abdominal circuit (1s) (using weights)

Hip Rotation: 10r (each side)

Hip roll: 15r

Knee Pull-in: 25r

Diagonal Sit-up: 12r

Russian Twist: 10r (each side); down in three sec, pause one sec, up at max speed

Weight: _____

Back Extension: 10r x 2s; up at moderate speed, no pause, down in four sec

Weight: _____

6. **Wrist-forearm circuit (2s) (using weights)** Week 1 40% Max; Week 2 50% Max; Week 3 60% Max; Week 4 70% Max

    Wrist Curls: Flexors: 20r; moderate speed

        Weight: _____

    Wrist Curls: Extension: 20r; moderate speed

        Weight: _____

    Forearm Pronation: 20r; moderate speed

        Weight: _____

    Forearm Supination: 20r; moderate speed

        Weight: _____

    Ulnar Deviation: 20r; moderate speed

        Weight: _____

    Radial Deviation: 20r; moderate speed

        Weight: _____

7. **Rotator-cuff circuit (2s) (using weights or tubing)**

    External Shoulder Rotation: 20r; moderate speed

        Weight: _____

    Internal Shoulder Rotation: 20r; moderate speed

        Weight: _____

    External Shoulder Rotation
    with Abduction: 20r; moderate speed

        Weight: _____

Additional work: Post-workout stretches

Supplementary aerobics: Week 4–8 (see chapter five)
Aerobic Training
Frequency: three sessions per week at intensity or 65 to 75% MHR for 20 minutes
Mode: Vary mode each time you work out. Choose from treadmill walking/running, stationary bike, stair climbing, or aerobic riding.

Precompetitive Phase

Block 2: Day 3

Note: Unless otherwise stated, rest one minute after every set; r=reps; s=sets; sec=seconds.

1. **Standard warm-up**

2. **Weight training (conventional method) (2s)** Week 1 60% Max; Week 2 65% Max; Week 3 70% Max; Week 4 75% Max

   Leg Press: 10r; up at max speed, pause for
                                 one second, down in three sec

   Weight: _____

   Back Extension: 10r; up at max speed, pause for
                                 one second, down in three sec

   Weight: _____

   Lat Pulldown: 10r; up at max speed, pause for
                                 one second, down in three sec

   Weight: _____

   Front Raises: 10r; up at max speed, pause for
                                 one second, down in three sec

   Weight: _____

   External Shoulder Rotations: 10–15r; moderate speed

   Weight: _____

Rest two to three minutes after each set

3. **Plyometrics and medicine ball**

   Chest Pass: 15r x 3s

   Weight: _____

Woodchops or Side Throws: 15r x 2s

    Weight: _____

4. **Abdominal circuit (2s) (using weights)**

Crossover Crunch:	25r (each side)
Seated Trunk Circles:	15r
Reverse Sit-up:	25r
Diagonal Sit-up:	12r
Russian Twist:	10r (each side); down in three sec, pause one sec, up at max speed

    Weight: _____

5. **Wrist-forearm circuit (1s) (using weights)** Week 1 40% Max; Week 2 50% Max; Week 3 60% Max; Week 4 70% Max

Wrist Curls: Flexors: 20r; moderate speed

    Weight: _____

Wrist Curls: Extension: 20r; moderate speed

    Weight: _____

Forearm Pronation: 20r; moderate speed

    Weight: _____

Forearm Supination: 20r; moderate speed

    Weight: _____

Ulnar Deviation: 20r; moderate speed

    Weight: _____

Radial Deviation: 20r; moderate speed

    Weight: _____

6. **Rotator-cuff circuit (2s)** Maximum weight of 5 lbs.

    External Shoulder Rotation: 20r; moderate speed

        Weight: _____

    Internal Shoulder Rotation: 20r; moderate speed

        Weight: _____

    External Shoulder Rotation
    with Abduction: 20r; moderate speed

        Weight: _____

Additional work: Post-workout stretches

Supplementary aerobics: Week 4–8 (see chapter five)
Aerobic Training
Frequency: three sessions per week at intensity or 65 to 75%
   MHR for 20 minutes
Mode: Vary mode each time you work out. Choose from
   treadmill walking/running, stationary bike, stair climbing,
   or aerobic riding.

Block 3: Peaking Phase Workouts

You should perform Block 3 workouts at least two but preferably three days a week for the first four weeks of the Golfer's
Stroke-Saver Workout. If you train three days per week, the
workouts for Days 1 and 3 are the same.

Note: A complex is a type of set in which two exercises are
performed alternately (instead of in the conventional method
of performing all sets of one exercise before moving to the next
exercise). A circuit is a set in which several exercises are
performed in sequence.

    After every workout you need to perform five to ten min-
utes of the post-workout stretches from chapter three.

    Also, you will supplement your Block 3 workouts with aer-
obic training performed preferably on the days you are resting
from the workouts.

Block 3: Peaking Phase Workouts

Duration: four weeks
Workouts: three per week using training components
  from chapter four

Supplementary Work
Aerobic training from chapter five

Peaking Phase

Block 3: Day 1

Note: Unless otherwise stated, rest one minute after every set;
  r=reps; s=sets; sec=seconds.

1. **Standard warm-up**

2. **Power circuit 1 (2s)** Week 1 70% Max; Week 2 75% Max;
   Week 3 80% Max; week 4 85% Max

Chest Press:	8r; down in two sec, no pause, up at max speed
Weight: _____	
Chest Pass	10r
Woodchops or Side Throws:	12r

Rest two to three minutes after each set

3. **Power complex (2s)**

Lat Pulldown:	8r; down in three sec, up at max speed, no pause
Weight: _____	
Pullover Toss:	8r
Weight: _____	

Rest two to three minutes after each set

4. **Weight training (conventional method) (2s)** Week 1 70% Max; Week 2 75% Max; Week 3 80% Max; Week 4 85% Max

| Side Lunge: | 4r (each side); down in two sec, no pause, up at max speed |

Weight: _____

| Pulldown: | 5r; down at max speed, no pause, up in two sec |

Weight: _____

| Back Extension: | 5r; up at max speed, no pause, down in two sec |

Weight: _____

5. **Abdominal circuit (2s)**

Reverse Sit-ups:	25r
Hip Raises:	20r
Crossover Crunch:	30r
Hip Rotation:	12r

6. **Wrist-forearm circuit (1s) (using weights)** Week 1 40% Max; Week 2 50% Max; Week 3 60% Max; Week 4 70% Max

| Wrist Curls: Flexors: | 20r; moderate speed |

Weight: _____

| Wrist Curls: Extension: | 20r; moderate speed |

Weight: _____

| Forearm Pronation: | 20r; moderate speed |

Weight: _____

| Forearm Supination: | 20r; moderate speed |

Weight: _____

Ulnar Deviation: 20r; moderate speed

   Weight: _____

Radial Deviation: 20r; moderate speed

   Weight: _____

7. **Rotator-cuff circuit (2s) (using weights or tubing)**

External Shoulder Rotation: 20r; moderate speed

   Weight: _____

Internal Shoulder Rotation: 20r; moderate speed

   Weight: _____

External Shoulder Rotation
with Abduction: 20r; moderate speed

   Weight: _____

Additional work: Post-workout stretches

Supplementary aerobics: Week 9–12 (see chapter five)
Aerobic Training
Frequency: three sessions per week at intensity or 65 to 75%
MHR for 20 minutes
Mode: Vary mode each time you work out. Choose from
treadmill walking/running, stationary bike, stair climbing,
or aerobic riding.

Peaking Phase

Block 3: Day 2

Note: Unless otherwise stated, rest one minute after every set; r=reps; s=sets; sec=seconds.

1. **Standard warm-up**

2. **Power complex 1 (3s)**

   Lat Pulldown: 8r

   Weight: _____

   Standing Trunk Twist: 8r

   Weight: _____

Rest two to three minutes after each set

3. **Weight training circuit (3s)**

   Squat: 8r; down in two sec, no pause, up at max speed

   Weight: _____

   Seated Row: 8r; up in two sec, no pause, down in two sec

   Weight: _____

   Calf raise (single leg):   12r; up at max speed, no pause, down in two sec

   Weight: _____

Rest two to three minutes after each set

4. Abdominal circuit 2s)

Crossover Crunch:	15r
Hip Raises:	20r
Reverse Sit-up:	30r
Seated Trunk Circles:	12r

5. Wrist-forearm circuit (1s) (using weights) Week 1 40% Max; Week 2 50% Max; Week 3 60% Max; Week 4 70% Max

Wrist Curls: Flexors: 20r; moderate speed
   Weight: _____

Wrist Curls: Extension: 20r; moderate speed
   Weight: _____

Forearm Pronation: 20r; moderate speed
   Weight: _____

Forearm Supination: 20r; moderate speed
   Weight: _____

Ulnar Deviation: 20r; moderate speed
   Weight: _____

Radial Deviation: 20r; moderate speed
   Weight: _____

6. Rotator-Cuff Circuit (2s) (using weights or tubing)

External Shoulder Rotation: 20r; moderate speed
   Weight: _____

Internal Shoulder Rotation: 20r; moderate speed
   Weight: _____

External Shoulder Rotation
with Abduction: 20r; moderate speed
   Weight: _____

Additional work: Post-workout stretches

Supplementary aerobics: Week 9–12 (see chapter five)
Aerobic Training
Frequency: three sessions per week at intensity or 65 to 75%
  MHR for 20 minutes
Mode: Vary mode each time you work out. Choose from
  treadmill walking/running, stationary bike, stair climbing,
  or aerobic riding.

Peaking Phase

Block 3: Day 3

Note: Unless otherwise stated, rest one minute after every set;
  r=reps; s=sets; sec=seconds.

1. **Standard warm-up**

2. **Power circuit 1 (2s)**

| Chest press: | 8r; down in two sec, no pause, up at max speed |

  Weight: _____

| Chest Pass: | 10r |
| Woodchops or Side Throws: | 12r |

Rest two to three minutes after each set

3. **Power complex (2s)**

| Lat Pulldown: | 8r; down in three sec, up at max speed, no pause |

  Weight: _____

| Pullover toss: | 8r |
  Weight: _____

Rest two to three minutes after each set

4. Weight training (conventional method) (2s)

Side Lunge:	4r (each side); down in two sec, no pause, up at max speed
Weight: _____	
Lat Pulldown:	5r; down at max speed, no pause, up in two sec
Weight: _____	
Back Extension:	5r; up at max speed, no pause, down in two sec
Weight: _____	

5. Abdominal circuit (2s)

Reverse Sit-ups:	25r
Hip Raises:	20r
Crossover Crunch:	30r
Hip Rotation:	12r

6. Wrist-forearm circuit (1s) (using weights) Week 1 40% Max; Week 2 50% Max; Week 3 60% Max; Week 4 70% Max

Wrist Curls: Flexors:	20r; moderate speed
Weight: _____	
Wrist Curls: Extension:	20r; moderate speed
Weight: _____	
Forearm Pronation:	20r; moderate speed
Weight: _____	
Forearm Supination:	20r; moderate speed
Weight: _____	
Ulnar Deviation:	20r; moderate speed
Weight: _____	
Radial Deviation:	20r; moderate speed
Weight: _____	

7. Rotator-Cuff Circuit (2s) (using weights or tubing)

External Shoulder Rotation: 20r; moderate speed

    Weight: _____

Internal Shoulder Rotation: 20r; moderate speed

    Weight: _____

External Shoulder Rotation
with Abduction: 20r; moderate speed

    Weight: _____

Additional work: Post-workout stretches

Supplementary aerobics: Week 9–12 (see chapter five)
Aerobic Training
Frequency: three sessions per week at intensity or 65 to 75%
    MHR for 20 minutes
Mode: Vary mode each time you work out. Choose from
    treadmill walking/running, stationary bike, stair climbing,
    or aerobic riding.

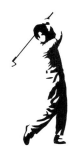

CHAPTER SEVEN

Eating for Eagles:
Golf-specific Nutrition Plan

When people look to the sports world for the best-conditioned athletes, they hardly think to look at golf. Take a look at some of the game's more visible players and you might understand why golfers are not held up as prime examples of great conditioning. While football, basketball, soccer, and hockey require—to differing degrees—brute strength, speed, and great stamina, all golfers seem to need is a powerful swing or a great putting stroke. Because golf consists of long periods of low-intensity action, with a few moments of great action, casual observers and some players think that golfers do not need to be fit to be good at the game. However, to be the best you need a complete conditioning program.

Complete conditioning, including sound nutrition, helps make golfers better. Proper nutrition benefits players of all abilities and helps take the natural athlete to the next level. The vast majority of golfers simply cannot reach their full potential unless they eat right. Proper nutrition enables the body to make gains in size, strength, endurance, and conditioning. All the practice in the world will only take you part of the way to improving your complete game. The rest depends on how well you fuel your body to perform.

Food fuels the body with energy. Highly skilled and highly trained athlete's such as pro golfers require high-performance nutrients, which include the right mix of fluids, carbohydrates, proteins, and fats.

Fluids

Golf is a game played in warm weather. Warm climates mean that golfers can lose more fluids through sweating than those who play cool-weather sports. When lost fluids are not replaced, the body temperature rises. This usually causes fatigue to set in more quickly, decreased performance quality, and a greater risk of heat injury. For these reasons, fluid intake is as needed as a club and balls.

Dehydration can be avoided by replenishing your body regularly with water *before* the onset of thirst. If you wait until you are thirsty, you have waited too long. By consuming fluids, you improve your performance by supplying your muscles with enough water for maximum muscle output. Cool water is best. Water between 40 and 50 degrees will be absorbed the fastest with less risk of cramping. The average person needs 64 ounces of water a day to maintain normal body functions. The well-trained golfer needs 96 to 128 ounces a day. Consuming 12 to 14 eight-ounce glasses of water per day is a good practice to follow both in-season and off-season. Eating plenty of fruits and vegetables at meals and as snacks will also help replace fluids and electrolytes, minerals, vitamins, and fiber, all of which are very important to your overall health.

Avoid fluids such as coffee, tea, and caffeinated soft drinks, which act as diuretics, dehydrating the body and robbing it of precious nutrients. Avoid alcohol, which dehydrates you and inhibits your performance. Sports drinks and juices provide water and are good sources of additional vitamins and carbohydrates, but they tend to be more filling and can lead to less frequent intake. Water is the fluid of choice. For proper hydration before a game or workout, drink two and a half cups of water two hours beforehand and another one and a half cups 15 minutes before the practice or game begins. Remember, you will need another eight to ten eight-once glasses a day on top of this.

Carbohydrates

Many consider carbohydrates the master fuel. For generating energy during practices and competition, they are the fuel of choice. The body breaks down carbohydrates into glycogen, which directly supplies fuel to your muscles. The calories carbohydrates contain are also quickly and efficiently burned during exercise. Researchers agree that golfers should keep their carbohydrate intake at 55 to 60 percent of their total calories.

There are two types of carbohydrates: simple and complex. Complex carbohydrates provide a slow and steady release of energy over a long period of time. Simple carbohydrates offer a quick but temporary rush of energy followed by low blood sugar, which robs you of overall energy, decreases concentration, and decreases performance intensity. Ideally, eat complex carbohydrates, which are found in fruits, root vegetables, beans, pasta, rice, grain breads, and cereals. Some sources of high levels of carbohydrates are:

Breakfast	Lunch/dinner	Dessert/snack
hot/cold cereal	pasta with sauce	angel food cake
pancakes/waffles	vegetables	pudding
muffins	bread/rolls	oatmeal raisin cookies
toast/English muffin	potato/rice/beans	sherbet
fruit/fruit juices	fruit juices	frozen yogurt

Protein

Protein used to be synonymous with red meat. Today, the trend toward low-fat diets has shed light on the many other excellent sources of protein. For a golfer, protein should account for 15 to 20 percent of total calories.

Beef, pork, lamb, poultry, and fish are excellent animal sources of complete protein. Complete protein means that 90 to 95 percent of the protein is absorbed by the body. Try to eat only lean meats, not cuts that are high in fat. Grains, nuts, beans, and tofu are also good sources of protein, but only 75 percent of these proteins are absorbed by the body. By limiting the amount of animal products consumed and including sources such as beans and dairy products in your diet, you should easily meet your daily protein requirement. Some sources of complete proteins are:

Meat	Fish	Dairy
beef	haddock	cheese
chicken	salmon	eggs
ham	tuna	milk
turkey	flounder	yogurt

Fats

Despite the bad press fat receives, it does have an important role—as a source of concentrated energy—in the golfer's diet. Although carbohydrate energy will be the first fuel your body uses during activity, you rely on energy from fat once the glycogen stores have been depleted. Glycogen is usually used up after 30 minutes of strenuous activity. Since golf rarely requires 30 minutes of straight activity, glycogen is the major fuel used in golf.

Limit your fat consumption to 15 percent of your total calories. Although fate does play a dietary role, too many fatty foods will likely lead to unnecessary and unwanted weight gain. Almost all fuels contain some fat, but try to avoid high-fat sources such as fried foods, candy, potato chips, doughnuts, cookies, dairy products (whole milk, cheese, cream, butter, ice cream), mayonnaise, and red meats. There are several ways of lowering your fat intake without reducing taste or substance:

- Prepare foods by broiling, baking, steaming, or poaching rather than frying.
- Remove skin from poultry and fish.
- Drink skim milk or water instead of whole milk.
- Substitute fish and white meat chicken for red meats.
- Avoid foods packed in oil.

Again, you don't want to eliminate fat completely from your diet, but it's best to keep your intake below 20 percent of your daily calories.

What to Eat When Dining out

When eating away from home you can still make healthy choices. In general, fast food is high in fat and low in nutrients so you need to be careful when picking from the menu. Here are some suggestions for several popular fast food restaurants:

	Breakfast	Lunch/dinner
McDonald's	Scrambled eggs English muffin with 　strawberry jam orange juice	two chicken sandwiches side salad with low calorie 　dressing 2% milk
Hardee's	hotcakes with 　butter and syrup English muffin 　with strawberry jam	two chicken breast 　sandwiches, no mayonnaise
Arby's		two junior roast beef 　sandwiches with lettuce 　and tomato 2% Milk
Taco Bell		two tacos two plain tortillas one bean burrito 2% milk
Pizza Hut		large spaghetti with meat 　sauce breadsticks 2% milk medium cheese pizza breadsticks 2% milk

Additional Eating Out Choices

Here are a few more basic guidelines to remember when you eat out. With a few adjustments you can eat out almost anywhere and follow this program. Listed are examples from different types of restaurants:

Continental (European Cuisine)

Most continental cuisine can be very balanced. Limit or avoid bread. Choose a grilled piece of protein with vegetables, a small serving of starchy carbohydrate, and a green salad.

Continental Meal Examples:

- Grilled fish or chicken with a small Caesar salad
- Grilled chicken breast or fish
- Vegetables, steamed
- Choose only one starch with your meal. If you are having bread pass on the potatoes, rice or pasta and ask for extra vegetables.
- Caesar salad
- Mineral water with lemon
- Gourmet pizza: Have a small, thin-crust gourmet pizza with grilled chicken and vegetables plus a large dinner salad. The pizza crust contains sufficient carbohydrates, so avoid any additional bread or dessert.

Italian

Choose a lean protein entree with vegetables and a salad. Include a small side order of pasta served with a tomato-based sauce and skip the bread.

Italian Meal Example
Lemon Chicken with Tomato Fettuccine
- Lemon Chicken
- Fettuccine with red sauce

- Vegetables
- Dinner salad with olive oil and vinegar dressing
- Mineral water

Japanese

Japanes cuisine is one of the most balanced choices, but watch out for eating too much rice and not getting enough protein. Avoid batter-fried tempura and choose grilled fish or chicken with vegetable and a small amount of steamed rice.

Japanese Meal Example
Grilled Teriyaki Chicken with Steamed Vegetables

- Teriyaki chicken
- Steamed vegetables
- Rice ($\frac{1}{2}$ to 1 cup)
- Small salad
- Hot tea

Chinese

Chinese cuisine can be very high in fat, sodium, and carbohydrates. The best choices are grilled or stir-fried chicken or fish with steamed vegetables and limited quantities of rice.

Chinese Meal Example
Stir-Fried Chicken and Broccoli

- Chicken
- Rice ($\frac{1}{2}$ to 1 cup)
- Broccoli
- Hot and sour soup
- Hot tea
- Water
- 1 fortune cookie

Deli

Delis generally provide quality protein but can be too high in fat. Choose a lean protein sandwich without cheese and use mayonnaise sparingly. Skip the potato and pasta salads that are loaded with fat and carbohydrates, and have a small piece of fruit or a side salad or cole slaw.

Deli Meal Example

Turkey on Rye

- Sliced turkey breast (3–4 ozs.)
- Two slices of rye or sourdough bread
- Lettuce and tomato
- Mayonnaise (use sparingly) and/or mustard
- 1 dill pickle
- 1 small piece of fruit or slaw
- Mineral water, iced tead, or diet soda

Pre- and Post-Event Meals

Pre- and post-workout, practice, or game nutrition is very important. You should eat two to four hours before your activity. This meal can prevent your blood sugar from getting too low, which can cause fatigue, dizziness, and lack of focus, and permits the absorption of carbohydrates as glycogen for optimal fuel use during exercise. Avoid overeating by eating only enough to fill your stomach to avoid hunger.

Before games, avoid foods with high cellulose content, such as lettuce, as they are hard to digest and can cause stomach irritation. Avoid spicy and fatty foods for the same reason. Too much protein and sugar intake can lead to dehydration and should be limited in pre-event meals. Liquids should be low in fat content and easily absorbed. Water is the best choice, but skim milk is also a good choice. Fruit juices can have a mild laxative effect, which may cause discomfort during your round. Don't drink beverages that contain caffeine because they act as diuretics and may increase pre-round nervousness. Whether it is breakfast, lunch, or dinner, stick with a high-carbohydrate pre- round or workout meal.

Post-event nutrition is as important as pre-event nutrition. Eat your post-game or post-practice meal as soon as possible to replenish carbohydrates and nutrients your body burned during activity. Ideally, you should eat no later than 60 to 90 minutes after the game, when your metabolism is at its highest. Your muscles are starving for nutritional replenishment at this time and recuperating muscles will absorb the highest amount of nutrients from food. After 90 minutes your metabolism begins to slow and tends to store food as fat instead of converting it into energy for muscles to store.

It is important to replace your body's fluids soon after a round or practice. Fruit, fruit juices, and high-carbohydrate sports drinks are good sources for quick carbohydrate and nutrient replacement.

Sample Tournament Menu

If you want to play great golf consistently, what you eat has an effect on your performance. Below is an eating plan for a day on the links. This plan will ensure you have optimum energy and power during your practice or round of golf—and this means better performance and lower scores.

Two hours prior to round:

Breakfast

5 scrambled egg whites
2 slices of whole wheat toast
sliced oranges and bananas
$2\frac{1}{2}$ cups of water

Pre-Round

$1\frac{1}{2}$ cups of water

Eat two hours into round to maintain energy.

Carry-along Lunch

1 16-ounce bottle of water
sandwich of sliced turkey breast and whole wheat bagel
   with mustard and or fat-free mayonnaise
1 piece of fruit

Eat three hours after lunch

Powerbar or ½ turkey sandwich
1 16-ounce bottle of water

Post-Round

1½ cups of water or sports drink

Dinner

4 ounces bluefin tuna
3 ounces dry long-grain brown rice
1 medium salad with low-fat dressing
2½ cups water

This combination of food will provide a steady supply of energy during your day and prevent the increased scores so common on the back nine.

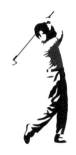

CHAPTER EIGHT

Designing a Training Program

Whether you are an elite professional golfer like Nancy Lopez or Mark O'Meara, or a serious recreational golfer trying to improve your game and conditioning level, one common obstacle stands in your way: time! How do you organize a training schedule to improve flexibility, aerobic conditioning, power, muscular strength, and endurance, and still play golf? That is what this book has covered thus far. The basic components are discussed; then sample programs for golfers are provided (see chapter six) and can be used as templates for designing an optimal program for your game.

What's the first step? Have a plan! An important aspect of designing a comprehensive training program is having a focused plan or set of goals. This is referred to as "needs analysis." No player, whether a professional player who has all day to devote to the game or a recreational player who has to balance family, work, and other responsibilities, has time to do all components of a training program every day.

In addition to time limitations, the body has its own limitations. To optimize the time you spend training for golf and minimize the risks of overtraining, such as burnout, fatigue, and injury, you must formulate a plan to prioritize and identify key areas of need.

One recommended way to formulate your plan is to use what the experts use—fitness testing. Chapter two provided groups of tests that you can do with little or no equipment to identify your skill or fitness level in the major categories of fitness: flexibility, strength, and aerobic conditioning.

Using testing to highlight the specific areas accomplishes two goals. First, you immediately know what area you need to work on, and second, you can gauge your improvement as you train. This means you will be able to update or change your program as you continue to train. Using the testing protocol and results provided in chapter two will provide you with an ideal start in designing your complete conditioning program and will highlight the areas you need to emphasize to improve your game and fitness levels.

Training Program Components

- **Individuality:** You should individualize a training program for your specific needs. Using the sport science–testing approach is one way of making a self-tailored program.

- **Specificity:** Adaptations the body makes to training are specific to the type of training or stresses that the body encounters. Therefore, your program should be golf-specific. Throughout this book, examples of how the body is stressed in golf are provided, and the training programs in chapter six are based on these stresses.

- **Overload and adaptation:** To enhance the body's strength or cardiovascular conditioning levels, we must apply and exercise stress or overload. An example of overloads in training programs would be using weights or running. The nature of the overload you use determines the type and degree of the body's adaptation response. We use overloads specific to golfers so the body will adapt in ways to enhance your golf performance.

- **Progression:** If you follow a program such as those in chapter six, the body will initially adapt to the loads and stresses of that program. However, if you do not increase the training, you will get no further gains or adaptations. Therefore, you must periodically increase your program so the body continues to improve and adapt to the new training loads.

- **Overtraining and recovery:** Overtraining occurs when the exercise overload is too stressful for the body to correctly adapt. Typical signs of overtraining are excessive fatigue, pain, emotional stress, and irritability and burnout. Overtraining does not just make you bored, it can make physiological improvements difficult, if not impossible. It produces tired, weak muscles, which at best will not grow and at worst will be at great risk for injury. To avoid overtraining you must increase training loads slowly, avoid heavy training on consecutive days, and use cross-training methods. Using recovery periods is the primary way of preventing overtraining. Athletes use a recovery period, sometimes hours, one day, or two weeks, to avoid tissue damage and overtraining, and to prevent burnout. Following a proper periodization schedule will ensure that recovery is part of your program.

Setting Realistic Goals

In chapter two you were presented with the fitness testing results using ranges from "excellent" to "needs improvement." As you can see in many categories, there are only small differences between "excellent," "average," or "needs improvement." The reason for this is that fitness improvements do not always come quickly or overnight, and many times involve small changes in time, speed, flexibility, and so on. Using these charts will guide you in setting realistic goals. Don't expect to improve from the "needs improvement" category to "excellent" in two weeks. Instead set small performance goals that you can attain incrementally as your training continues.

Be sure to set performance goals rather than outcome goals. An **outcome goal**, although attractive and inspiring, is not under your direct control and often is unattainable. An example of an outcome goal would be, "I will win the U.S. Open Championship." Obviously this goal is not under your control and does not consider performances of other players and other elements. An example of performance goals would be, "I will be able to do 15 push-ups in one minute," "I will improve my aerobic fitness level so I am not tired on the last four holes of my golf matches," and so on. **Performance goals** are under your control; they involve using goals that you set and train for.

Finally, allow enough time to attain your goals. Improvement in fitness levels cannot occur overnight. As you learned in chapter four, it takes a minimum of four to six weeks to adapt the muscles that affect strength and performance. Flexibility, if done properly, also comes gradually through a dedicated program of static stretching. Typically, you should not retest your fitness levels sooner than eight weeks or, in many cases, every three months to allow adaptations and improvements in training to occur.

Periodization Training

Another important concept related to fitness-program design is **periodization**. Periodization is a long-term training plan that systematically controls and changes volume, intensity, frequency, and duration of training and competition. Its purpose is to optimize performance at specific times and prevent overtraining, chronic fatigue, and burnout. The training volume relates to the amount of work you perform, the intensity refers to how hard you work in your training session, and the frequency measures how often you train. The duration relates to the length of your workout or training session.

Periodization has been used for decades in sports such as weightlifting, swimming, and track and field, but it also has benefits for golfers. Applying periodization to golf allows a player to integrate many types of training in several specific time periods or stages. Each stage within a periodization cycle has a specific goal and purpose and allows the player to work toward competitive events in a structured way.

Have you ever noticed that golf is one of the few sports without an off-season? If you want, you can play in a tournament every week. Competitions in sports such as basketball, baseball, and soccer occur at a specific time of year and their seasons end. Although there can be advantages to playing in many events, the problem with playing golf week after week is that you may risk injury, get stale, or even burn out.

What do many of the top professionals do to avoid these problems? They follow a carefully designed periodization training program. Each individual periodization training program is based on your fitness level and your planned tournament schedule. Therefore, at the beginning of the year (with your coach, if you have one) it is important to decide which tournaments are most important for your golf development. Start by testing yourself using the fitness tests in chapter two to determine your baseline fitness level and then proceed with training. A golf-specific periodization training program consists of four different phases: the preparation phase, the precompetitive phase, the competitive (peaking) phase, and the active rest (transition) phase.

Preparation Phase

It is important to develop a strong aerobic base in the Preparation Phase focusing on high-volume and low-intensity work. This means that, in addition to your golf practice you should focus on long-distance activities such as running, biking, or swimming for at least 20 minutes continuously. The length of this phase may vary but should not be shorter than four weeks.

The training components of the Preparation Phase include the following:

- Challenge the aerobic energy system, for example with 20 to 40 minutes of aerobic training at 70 to 85 percent of maximum heart rate three to four times per week.

- Establish a strength base, for example strength training using a high-repetition (10 to 15 repetitions per set, with two to three sets), low-resistance training program.

- Include technical and tactical training, for example on-course training that would incorporate changes in swing mechanics, develop new shots, and so on.

There is little golf-specific training in this phase. It emphasizes low resistance and high repetition to establish a fitness base. The later, more specific phases include lower work output and higher overall intensity.

Precompetitive Phase

In the Precompetitive Phase, training routines should become more golf specific, increasing the intensity while reducing the training volume. Although there will be an aerobic component to the training program, the focus should be more on explosive movement and strength-training exercises. Again, the length of this phase should be at least four weeks.

The second phase in the periodization cycle is the Precompetitive Phase. In this phase the intensity level increases and the theme becomes more golf specific.

- Improve speed and power, for example with club drills and plyometrics.
- Improve muscular strength, for example performing two to four sets with eight to ten repetitions, decreasing training volume and increasing the intensity of the resistance exercise.
- Maintain aerobic status, for example performing aerobic exercise two times per week for 20 to 30 minutes.
- Improve golf-specific skills, for example on-course training focuses on golf-specific drills, practice rounds, and simulated matches in preparation for competition.

Competitive (Peaking) Phase

Because athletes can sustain a true peak in performance for only three weeks, you should focus on maintaining muscular strength and endurance levels during the competitive, or peaking, phase. Train at high intensities while determining the volume by the number of rounds and tournaments in this period. Golfers usually terminate aerobic training and weight training during this phase. Some athletes may travel with rubber tubing and perform a light set or two of 10 to 15 repetitions to maintain strength in golf-specific areas, such as the rotator-cuff or forearms, but the primary focus during this time remains on peak performance.

The components of the Competitive (Peaking) Phase are:

- Peak performance!
- High-intensity workouts.
- Golf competition or golf-specific training.

Active Rest (Transition) Phase

During the early part of the Active Rest, or Transition, Phase, take some time to recover from golf. Maintain your fitness level by participating in other activities, such as basketball, soccer, running, hiking, swimming, and so on. As you start playing golf again, work on your swing technique. Depending on the time of year, this phase could last from one to four weeks. The goal in this phase is to rest from the physical and psychological stresses of training and competition.

The components of the Active Rest, or Transition, Phase are:

- Rest from golf.
- Cross-train to maintain fitness levels.
- Emphasize fun, low-intensity workouts.
- Rest one to four weeks.

Organizing a Periodized Program

Because most golfers' schedules do not contain an off-season, applying the periodized model to golf can be tricky. One way to structure the periodization cycle is to choose tournaments that carry the most significance and build the training phases based on the performance peaks. As an example, a player hoping to peak for the U.S. Open in late May would spend the four to six weeks before it in the Precompetitive Phase. The player would be in the Preparation Phase, doing aerobic training, building a strength base, and so on, in late winter/early spring.

One complete periodization cycle is termed a microcycle, in which the player goes through each phase one time. Groupings of microcycles are called a macrocycle, which often would contain an entire year's tournaments or performance schedule. Following each microcycle of periodization, players typically do fitness testing and needs analysis so the next training cycle can address specific weaknesses or injury-risk characteristics and improve performance.

Starting Your Program

Four principles may assist you in balancing the various elements of a training program and fitting them into an effective regimen successfully:

1. **Integrate flexibility training with all other aspects of your training.** There is usually not enough time for any golfer to spend an hour a day on stretching. However, if you integrate flexibility training before and after all other modes of training, then you usually won't require a specific block of time dedicated only to flexibility training. Additionally, a brief stretching period before and after a weight or aerobic workout is as important and accomplishes the same goals as stretching before and after your on-course training.

2. **Prioritize!** A golfer who simultaneously implements several components, such as strength training, aerobic conditioning, plyometrics, and so on into a start-up fitness program is bound to fail. Pick one or two components to focus on initially and build your program from that training focus to a more comprehensive program over time. An example would be adding a regimen of flexibility training before and after a round of golf, along with shoulder and trunk exercises for two to four weeks.

Then add items to the program, such as aerobic training. Begin with the one or two items that need the most emphasis and build the program as your body allows.

3. **Don't expect immediate results.** If you do you may be disappointed. As you learned in the chapter on strength training (chapter four), it takes a minimum of four to six weeks to change the muscle. Similarly, the program you initially develop may take several weeks to garner results; this is normal.

4. **More is not necessarily better. Remember to include rest and recovery.** When putting together a training program that includes several components, you cannot always perform every component every day. In many instances you can perform strength training two or three times per week, allowing the trained muscles to recover a day or two between sessions. The same would hold true for aerobic conditioning and other elements in the program.

In summary, I hope these principles will guide you in applying the individual concepts from the earlier chapters in this book. The sample workouts in chapter six are templates for you to use and modify based on individual needs. Whether you are Tiger Woods, Nancy Lopez, an aspiring junior competitive player, or a recreational player, adding a fitness program will enhance your performance level and increase your enjoyment of the game.

The End of the Beginning

You and I are old friends now. We've come a long way together. I must admit that I have enjoyed this opportunity to provide the guidelines you will use to become the best golfer you can through fitness training.

Now it's time for you to really get down to business!

You've learned how to test your beginning fitness level to create the shortest possible program.

You've learned how to warm-up and stretch in a manner that immediately improves your distance and decreases your score.

You've learned how to perform a brief 20-minute-interval aerobic program that boosts your stamina and still leaves you time to play golf.

You've learned how to fuel your body before, during, and after your round of golf to create a peak performance state.

You've learned how tour players combine all the elements of fitness in a powerful program that is short and to the point.

Yes, we have come a long way together!

Unlike other authorities, I haven't just packaged this information to create a book . . . but to launch a relationship. As you set out to implement these techniques and achieve your greater golf self, I want to know how you are doing. Thousands of people around the world regularly share their journeys with me. They tell me what's working, what's not, how they've perfected the techniques they learned from me, and what kind of additional information they require to reach their golf objectives.

I invite you to keep in touch and keep me informed about your progress. Moreover, I invite you to keep me as your secret success weapon. I know that success is not achieved by some effortless two-stepping. It's not inevitable. It's the result of continual deliberation and constant refinement. It's the product of thoughtfulness, persistence, unrelenting focus, and, yes, great humility and an ability to remain open to beneficial change when those around you succumb to the numbing idea of the "tried and true."

There will be days, even many days, as you implement and develop your training program that you will encounter the fate of all those who strive to be the best they can. People will ask why you are training this way—this strange way most people are unaware even exists.

All this you must take in stride. You are a champion and a superior person, the kind of person who must succeed.

When those days come, when things are not going your way, when you feel the training is too much for you, study this resource again. Familiarize yourself with the many tools I've created over the years. Finally, keep my e-mail address close at hand. It helps to know you have a friend, supporter, and fellow player just this close ready to listen to you, push, empathize, or exult, as the case may be. Please email me at askinnerjr@aol.com to keep me informed about how I can be of more help.

We're all in this together. And if I can help you achieve the promise of this book's title, I will. Just remember to share the joy of your achievement with me. After all, I know how very hard you've worked to earn it! Just remember, I'm only an e-mail away at askinnerjr@aol.com.

Index

* * *

Thank you for your purchase of this book. Not only are you improving your golf game but you are helping to cure breast and prostate cancer. I am donating 50 percent of my royalties from this project to the Susan G. Komen Fund for the awareness and cure of breast cancer and to CaP CURE, whose mission is to prevent and cure prostate cancer.

Below you will find out a little more about each organization and how to donate more if you would like to keep up the fight.

Prostate cancer is the second leading cause of death among men. CaP CURE is the world's largest private source of funding for prostate cancer research.

CaP CURE was founded in 1993 with an urgent mission: identify and support prostate-cancer research that will rapidly translate into treatments and cures. Together with survivors, scientists, and advocates, CaP CURE has established a system that encourages collaboration, reduces bureaucracy, and speeds the process of discovery.

CaP CURE reaches out to private industry, the patient advocacy community, and government research institutions. These partnerships provide a model to speed the cure for prostate cancer—and all cancers.

Contact information:

The Association for the Cure of Cancer of the Prostate (CaP CURE)
1250 Fourth Street, Suite 360
Santa Monica, CA 90401
1-800-757-CURE
1-310-458-2873
Fax: 1-310-458-8074
E-mail: capcure@capcure.org
Web site: www.Capcure.org

*   *   *

An estimated 211,300 new invasive cases of breast cancer are expected to occur among women in the United States during 2003. An estimated 39,800 women will die from breast cancer. It is estimated that 1,300 men will be diagnosed and 400 men will die of breast cancer during 2003. Breast cancer is the leading form of cancer among American women and is second only to lung cancer in cancer deaths. Breast cancer is the leading cause of cancer deaths among women ages 40–59.

The Susan G. Komen Foundation is a global leader in the fight against breast cancer through its support of innovative research and community-based outreach programs. Working through a network of U.S. and international affiliates and events like the Komen Race for the Cure®, the foundation is fighting to eradicate breast cancer as a life-threatening disease by funding research grants and supporting education, screening, and treatment projects in communities around the world.

Contact information:

    Susan G. Komen Breast Cancer Foundation
    5005 LBJ Freeway, Suite 250
    Dallas, TX 75244

To mail donations:

    P. O. Box 650309
    Dallas, TX 75265-0309
    Phone: 1-972-855-1600
    Fax: 1-972-855-1605
    Web site: www.komen.org